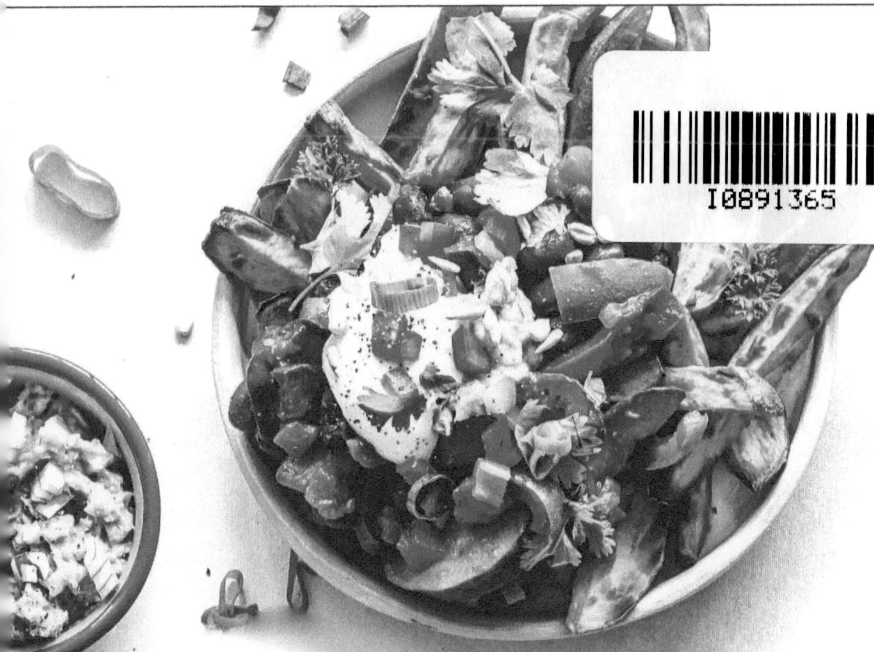

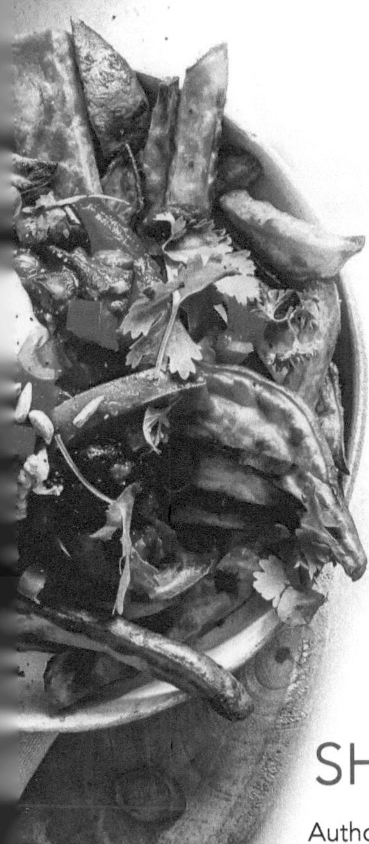

MINDFUL BITE JOYFUL LIFE

365 DAYS OF MINDFUL EATING

SHEILA H.FORMAN Ph.D.

Author of *TAME Your Appetite: The Art of Mindful Eating*

Mindful Bite, Joyful Life: 365 Days of Mindful Eating

Published by TVGuestpert Publishing

ISBN-13: 978-1-7358981-4-8
BISAC CODES: HEA006000, HEA017000, HEA010000

Nationwide Distribution through Ingram & New Leaf Distributing Company.

Front Book Cover Design by Lynn Pelkey
Book Design by Carole Allen Design Studio
Author headshots by Cathryn Farnsworth
Edited by TVGuestpert Publishing

11664 National Blvd, #345
Los Angeles, CA. 90064
310-584-1504
www.TVGuestpertPublishing.com
www.TVGuestpert.com
First Printing 2022
10 9 8 7 6 5 4 3 2 1

DISCLAIMER

The information, ideas and suggestions offered in this book are not intended as a substitute for professional advice. Before following any of the suggestions offered, you should confer with your medical and mental health professionals to make certain that the information is right for you. Neither the author nor the publisher shall be liable or responsible in any way for any loss or damage alleged to arise from the information contained herein.

In addition, throughout this book you will find "case studies." Each case study is a composite of various experiences presented for illustrative purposes only. Any resemblance to any person, dead or alive, is merely a coincidence.

A word about weight loss–mindful eating is a non-diet approach to weight management. It is not a diet or quick weight-loss program. Some people lose weight with this approach; others do not. Some initially gain weight when they abandon previous restrictions. The research on mindful eating says that the more you practice mindful eating techniques, especially mindfulness meditation, the greater the likelihood for sustainable weight loss. Because weight loss depends upon your own efforts, body type, and medical and psychiatric history, the author and publisher make no guarantees regarding weight loss.

Lastly, although Dr. Sheila Forman is licensed to practice psychology in the State of California, no psychotherapist–client relationship has been established by the information presented in this book, nor by any program or product Dr. Forman has created.

◆◆◆

DEDICATION

This journey into mindful eating is dedicated to my niece Lauren Elle Jacobowitz as she starts her journey to becoming a physician. Lauren's dedication to the medical profession and the healing she will provide in the future is an inspiration for me to keep doing what I am doing. With young people like Lauren at the helm, we are in store for a glorious future.

◆◆◆

Mindfulness is . . .

"paying Attention in the present moment, on purpose, non-judgmentally."

Jon Kabat-Zinn, PhD, in *Full Catastrophe Living*

TABLE OF CONTENTS

Introduction

Welcome to the world of mindful eating. Over the course of the next 365 days, I will guide you through the principles, tools, and techniques of mindful eating.

Taking your journey one day at a time will help establish mindful eating as a real habit and, in so doing, you will heal the disordered eating you may be struggling with, as well as extend wellness to other areas of your life.

You don't need to diet or do anything different than you are already doing except apply each day's teaching. Some days will be easy and others you may struggle with. That's okay because with a foundation of mindfulness there is no judgment or striving, only acceptance and moment-to-moment observations.

I recommend you start this book from the beginning even if it's the middle of the year because the teachings build upon each other. After you've done the course for a year, you can redo it starting with wherever you are in the calendar. Use the wisdom offered in this book as your guide to a new relationship with food. Use what feels right to you. Test the suggestions and make notes on your outcomes.

This book is written as a one-year journey because it takes time to change old habits, beliefs and thinking patterns. Give yourself the gift of a year. You will be amazed at what you can accomplish and the changes you will witness in the course of twelve months. I would love to hear from you so be sure to get onto my email list and join my Facebook page. You can also get my book, *Tame Your Appetite: The Art of Mindful Eating*, which goes into depth on a lot of concepts covered in this book. Although you do not have to read *Tame Your Appetite*, together they will make a difference to your relationship with food.

Here's to a great year, peace with food and mindful eating habits.

Dr. Sheila

365 Days of Mindful Eating

January

JANUARY 1:

MINDFUL EATING—IT ALL STARTS WITH AWARENESS

Welcome to the first day of your year's journey to become a mindful eater. Much of what you will read about and learn over these next 365 (or maybe 366!) days will reflect my own journey and those of the people to whom I have taught mindful eating. You will find as we move forward that this is in fact a journey. You will have great days and challenging days. Some of the habits I will be teaching you will come easily; others not so much. I suggest you keep a journal for these 365 days of your journey. Documenting your efforts will support you as you embrace a mindful way of life. Writing down what happens to you over the next year will help you stay the course, master mindful eating and apply mindfulness principles to your whole life.

As a result of becoming a mindful eater, I let go of the excess weight that had been yo-yoing on and off my body for my entire adult life. I am confident that those pounds are gone for good as long as I continue to practice my mindful eating habits and apply mindfulness to my life in general. I can't promise that you will have the same results—your results may in fact be even better—but what I can tell you is that the more your practice and apply mindful eating and mindfulness to your life, the healthier and happier you will become. By doing that, you can let go of your excess weight in a way and at a rate that is right for you. You'll understand what this means as we move along.

For today, we will begin with the definition of mindful eating.

Mindful eating is eating with awareness of your body's needs and preferences as well as your emotional states and desires.

Consider this definition and how embracing it may affect your weight, your body and your life. In your journal, reflect on this definition and what it might mean for your weight and food struggles. As we move along in this journey the meaning of each word in the definition will become clearer. For today, just start where you are and give yourself credit for being here.

***Today:* Reflect upon the definition of mindful eating and answer the journal question below.**

***Today's Journal Question:* How might mindful eating help you with your weight and food struggles?**

JANUARY 2:

ARE YOU A MINDLESS EATER?

If mindfulness is about awareness then everything you are unaware of can be deemed mindlessness. In fact, mindlessness means "being without awareness." So, in terms of eating behavior, mindless eating means eating without awareness and that is so much of the eating that we all do. Examples of mindless eating include getting popcorn every time you go to the movies simply because that's what you do. Or reaching the bottom of the popcorn bucket and being surprised that there's no more left. Mindless eating is also eating the entire portion that's placed in front of us regardless of whether we are hungry for it. It also means eating food as directed by some diet list or program regardless of whether you're in the mood for it or if it even tastes good. We may also be eating mindlessly when we choose the same foods over and over again without checking in with our body to see if that's really what it needs to be nourished. We are eating mindlessly when we reach for something out of habit, for example, every time you feel upset you have some ice cream.

Yesterday, I asked you to reflect on how mindful eating might help your weight loss efforts. Today I'd like you to reflect on your mindlessness. Where in your life are you mindless? In other words, where in your life are you acting strictly out of habit when that habit may no longer serve you? Because we're talking about eating on this journey, you can start with mindless eating. Where, what and when do you eat mindlessly? As you become a mindful eater you will find that being mindful will positively impact other areas your life as well. We'll talk more about that in the weeks and months ahead.

***Today:* Continue to reflect upon the definition of mindful eating from yesterday and begin today to notice (without judgment or strain) where you are being mindless.**

***Today's Journal Question:* Besides weight loss, what do you hope to get from mindful eating?**

JANUARY 3:
CULTIVATING INNER WISDOM

Inside each of us is an all-knowing wise self who understands who we are, what we need and what we don't. We experience this all-knowing wise self as that little voice deep inside that talks to us. Often it tells us things that we don't want to hear. That little voice is, what we call in the world of mindful eating, your Inner Wisdom.

An important part of developing mindful eating skills is identifying and listening to your Inner Wisdom. Learning to hear the voice inside your head and being willing to abide by it are worthwhile skills. Learning them will help you not only with eating and weight issues, but also with your life in general.

I'll give an example of what occurred for me recently. As I was preparing myself a snack, I was putting blackberries into a bowl in anticipation of adding some yogurt and almonds to it. This is one of my favorite snacks. I poured the container of blackberries into a strainer to rinse them. Typically, I would take this entire pile of berries and put it into a bowl with the yogurt and almonds. But as I looked at the berries in the bowl that voice inside my head said, "There are too many berries in the bowl today. You don't need so many." I heard it and I observed the number of berries in the bowl. I realized that in the past I would have eaten all of them because on the surface they seemed to be a reasonable amount.

However, because I am building my Inner Wisdom and I'm listening to my inner voice I recognized that my body was telling me that for this day, in this moment, with this snack those are just too many berries. So, I went to my cabinet and I pulled out a container. I divided the berries in half, leaving half in the bowl and putting the other half back into the refrigerator. As I did this, I felt a sense of satisfaction and pride. I also felt that I now had the right number of berries in the bowl for my snack. I proceeded to add the yogurt and the almonds and when I looked into the bowl it looked exactly like the right amount of food for my body at this moment in time.

In the past I would've eaten double the amount of berries. And while that might not sound like a crime, if I am trying to be mindful and addressing my body's needs, those extra berries, albeit a healthy choice, would have been more than what my body required. This time I chose to listen to and obey my Inner Wisdom. As I ate my snack, I found it to be especially delicious and satisfying.

For today, do the best you can to listen for that inner voice. You don't have to do what it says, just notice it. In other words, become aware of it. Listen to when it tells you your portion is too big or too small. Listen when it tells you that your choices are good or could be better. Each time you become aware of your inner voice you are strengthening your Inner Wisdom. In time, you will learn to listen to and abide by that wisdom but for now because we are building the skill of awareness, all you have do is simply notice it.

Today: **Listen for the still, inner voice that is trying to guide you to healthy choices and right action. Can you hear it? What is it saying?**

Today's Journal Question: **How in touch are you with your Inner Wisdom?**

JANUARY 4:

ONE-MINUTE MEDITATION

At the heart of mindful eating is mindfulness meditation. Now before you get all freaked out and worried about the idea of meditating, let me assure you meditation is probably not what you think it is. In fact, mindfulness-based meditation may surprise you. If mindfulness is about awareness then I bet you can guess that mindfulness meditation is about becoming aware of your mind. It's about noticing what you mind is doing. Is it thinking? Planning? Rehearsing? Repeating? Worrying?

By spending time with your mind each day, you will become better able to notice where it's going and what it's doing. As your awareness of your mind increases so will your awareness of everything else. Eventually that will naturally translate into being more aware of your food and eating habits. Awareness, as you will come to experience, creates the opportunity for change. And change is what we are moving towards. To begin your meditation practice, simply do the following:

- Find a comfortable place to sit or lie down.
- Loosen any tight-fitting clothing or shoes.
- Close your eyes.
- Take deep breath in through your nose and then exhale through your mouth.
- Focus your attention on your breath and continue breathing for one minute.
- If your mind wanders, and it probably will, simply notice that it has done so and turn your attention back to your breath.
- After a minute you can open your eyes and go back to your day or you can continue longer if you so desire.

Congratulations, you have just meditated. Practice this one-minute meditation once a day beginning today. If you miss a day, no worries, simply start again.

***Today:* Meditate for one minute.**

***Today's Journal Question:* What is your reaction to the description of mindfulness meditation and your first experience of meditating?**

JANUARY 5:
EAT ONE BITE MINDFULLY

If you have taken a mindfulness meditation class you may have been introduced to the famous raisin experiment. That experiment has you eating a single raisin slowly, mindfully. I use the raisin experiment in all my TAME Your Appetite programs. The purpose of that experiment is to teach you what mindful eating is all about. To introduce you to mindful eating today I would like you to eat a raisin mindfully. If you don't like raisins choose another morsel of food to do this experiment. What does eating mindfully mean? It means selecting one raisin (morsel of food) and doing the following:

- Put raisin (or morsel of food) on a fork, spoon or between your fingers.
- Look at it. Notice its colors and textures.
- Bring it to your nose and sniff. Notice its scent.
- Touch it to your lips. Feel its texture.
- Place it in your mouth, but don't chew. Feel it. Roll it over your tongue.
- Bite into it. Notice its flavor.
- Chew it but don't swallow.
- Now swallow and feel the food slip down your throat.
- Place your hand on your stomach and imagine the bite of food settling there.

That's it. You just ate mindfully! Please know that as you move forward with mindful eating you won't be eating every bite like this. But getting started with a single bite like this each day will help you get the hang of it.

Today: **Eat one bite of food mindfully and meditate for one minute.**

Today's Journal Question: **How would you describe your experience of eating one bite of food in the manner described above?**

JANUARY 6:

WHAT ABOUT THE SCALE?

Most people come to mindful eating to lose weight and weight loss is a natural by-product, but it is not the focus. Weighing oneself is an important part of this process because it provides information on what is working and what needs work. But focusing on the number on the scale can be counterproductive. For our purposes, a weekly weigh-in is sufficient to gather information on your progress without getting too hung up on results. You can also choose not to weigh yourself at all. Or weigh yourself less frequently, perhaps once a month. It's up to you. But I strongly recommend that you do not weigh yourself more than once a week.

When you get on the scale tell yourself that part of learning to eat mindfully is learning to accept "what is" without judgment. The number on the scale is purely information for your use and benefit and not something with which to judge yourself (positively or negatively).

Your "goal," if you want to call it that, is to allow your body to reach the weight that is right for it using the guidance mindful eating provides. Should that number be higher or lower than the number you have in mind, so be it. Choose to trust your body's wisdom and this mindful eating journey.

Today: **Weigh yourself if you like but then don't weigh yourself again for at least another week. Continue to eat one bite of food mindfully and meditate for one minute.**

Today's Journal Question: **What has your relationship been with the scale?**

JANUARY 7:

I CAN'T BELIEVE I ATE THE WHOLE THING!

If you are anywhere near my age, you might remember the old Alka-Seltzer commercials with the phrase, "I can't believe I ate the whole thing!" Alka-Seltzer, you may know, is a remedy for indigestion. So is mindfulness. Being mindful and developing Inner Wisdom is, in part, about knowing how certain foods, certain amounts, and certain combinations affect you. Foods you may think you love may not love you back. Being mindful means noticing when the foods you eat or the drinks you drink don't agree with you and then making a thoughtful, mindful decision about whether to consume it again.

Let me give you an example. Sometimes on Sunday mornings I like to enjoy an English muffin topped with cream cheese and lox. Such a breakfast is a real treat for me. Typically, I prepare half an English muffin and maybe add a few cherry tomatoes to the plate. One Sunday morning I awoke feeling a bit hungrier than usual. I prepared my special breakfast but this morning I did not have any cherry tomatoes (forgot to put them on the shopping list – a mindless moment!) so I decided to have the whole English muffin topped with cream cheese and lox. I sat down to eat my breakfast and everything tasted delicious. I was at the moment happy with my choice. But that all changed about an hour later when I noticed that I was not feeling well. I felt a bit of heartburn. I was also burping a bit (sorry for the graphic description, but I think it's valuable to share this). I felt as if my breakfast had not made it all the way down to my stomach but rather was stuck somewhere mid-chest. I took out my journal and made some notes about this.

I realized that a half serving of this special breakfast served my body well but for some reason a full serving did not. My gastrointestinal distress was my body's way of communicating its Inner Wisdom to me. As I "listened" I understood that a smaller version of this breakfast is best for me. Going forward I will keep this information in mind so that I can make an informed, mindful decision next Sunday should I choose to treat myself again.

Do the foods you choose agree with you? Are you ignoring your body's signals that something is not right because you want to keep eating? Being mindful means being aware of how food and drinks affect you—good and bad. Pay attention to whether your favorite foods are also your body's favorites or if you need to make some adjustments. Sometimes less is more as is in my case. Other times, out of sight might be the best way to go. You decide . . . mindfully.

***Today:* Pay attention to how your body reacts to the foods you eat. Continue eating one bite of food mindfully and meditating for one minute.**

***Today's Journal Question:* How does your body communicate with you when it likes or dislikes something you have consumed?**

JANUARY 8:
WHAT IF . . . ?

When I first started studying mindful eating, I received training in Mindfulness-based Eating Awareness (MB-EAT). During this training, Dr. Jean Kristeller, the founder of MB-EAT, asked, "What if a year from now you lost weight, maybe not as much as you'd like, but you were more in control of your life and eating, and the weight you lost felt permanent because it reflected change that you could live with for the rest of your life. . . . ?" What if . . . ? My immediate thought was "how wonderful!" So often people come to me wanting to lose weight and lose it now! I explain to them that taking a non-diet approach takes longer but has the potential for longer-lasting results. I explain that by addressing the underlying thoughts, feelings and behaviors that led them to gain and hold onto excess weight their weight will come off, but in my experience weight loss is the last piece to change. They are not happy with that information. But, when I pose that question to them, their perspective changes and we get to work. Ask yourself this same question and be honest with your answer. So many dieters are either at the same weight or heavier a year after they tried to lose weight. What if instead you were slimmer? What if . . . ?

***Today:* Eat one bite of food mindfully and meditate for one minute.**

***Today's Journal Question:* Answer Dr. Kristeller's question for yourself—"What if a year from now you lost weight, maybe not as much as you'd like, but you were more in control of your life and eating and the weight you lost felt permanent because it reflected change you could live with for the rest of your life?"**

JANUARY 9:
WHAT COLOR WAS YOUR LUNCH?

Here's a quick exercise for you to try. Take a moment and try to imagine the lunch you ate yesterday. First question, do you remember eating lunch yesterday? Second question, do you remember what you ate yesterday? If you don't remember, don't worry. Many people don't remember what they eat from day to day unless they are either following a diet plan that prescribes their daily food intake or they keep a food diary. Not remembering is part of mindlessness and will change as you keep on developing your mindful eating skills.

If you did remember what you ate for lunch yesterday, try to see your meal in your mind's eye. See the food on the plate, bowl or container. Remember where you were when you ate it. Now, remember what it looked like and ask yourself what colors were present. That's right, what colors? For example, yesterday I had blueberries with Greek yogurt and almonds. The colors in my bowl were purple, white, and golden brown. The bowl was also white and I used a silver spoon. The day before I had a chopped Cobb salad with crackers. That lunch had a rainbow of colors including green, white, yellow, red, brown, blue and orange.

It may seem silly to you to think about the colors in your lunch but doing so helps us be more present with our food and helps us appreciate it more. Having gratitude for our food and expressing gratitude towards those who contributed to the creation of our meal is part of mindful eating. We will do a gratitude exercise later on.

For today, take a moment and notice the colors in the next portion of food you eat. Even if it's only one color – let's say yellow because you are eating corn chips – notice the subtle differences in the color within the portion. No two corn chips will be exactly alike. If you add salsa to the chips, admire the bright red of the tomatoes and the green from the chili peppers. Using our eyes to see the food we are eating is a step towards mindful eating. They say beauty is in the eye of the beholder. I say beauty is on the plate in front of us.

***Today:* Notice the colors of the food you eat and continue to eat one bite of food mindfully and meditate for one minute.**

***Today's Journal Question:* How might really looking at your food affect your eating habits?**

JANUARY 10:
TAKE A FOOD SELFIE

I love to travel, and when I travel, I love to sample local cuisine. I also love to photograph it. In fact, if you look at any of my travel albums, they are equal parts historical monuments and food. When I'm traveling and I'm sampling local cuisine I take the time to admire the food and I savor it.

What I know now that I didn't know before is that in doing so, I was eating mindfully, and, as a consequence, I enjoyed the food more and was satisfied with the portions served. If you travel at all, you know that the portions served outside the United States are significantly smaller than what we are accustomed to and yet I was always satisfied and full from the smaller portions. Now I understand why.

Admiring the food, appreciating its authenticity, and savoring each and every bite because I knew it was unlikely I would ever eat it again led to increased satisfaction and pleasure.

So, whether it was goulash in Hungary, Pad Thai in Thailand or Wurst in Germany, I savored the delicacies offered. You can do the same thing without ever leaving the comfort of your home.

For today, take a photograph of something that you're about to eat before you eat it. Look at the photograph and ask yourself (1) does this food look appetizing? (2) is this food that I genuinely want to eat or is it something that I'm eating because it's available or prescribed? and (3) would I be happy sharing this photograph with someone else? Taking a photograph of your food and then looking at it before eating is another step towards mindfulness.

If you'd like, you can share your photographs on our Facebook page or Instagram. I'd love to see what you've been mindfully eating.

***Today:* Photograph your food and post it for our community to see. Continue to eat one bite of food mindfully and meditate for one minute.**

***Today's Journal Question:* What experiences do you have with food when you travel?**

JANUARY 11:
THREE-MINUTE MEDITATION

It's time to increase your daily meditation practice. Three minutes may not seem like a lot but it is a great way to incrementally establish your daily meditation practice. You've been doing one minute for the past week so three minutes should be a breeze. Simply do what you have been doing and just extend it by two minutes. If you have been struggling to find one minute to meditate each day, then start with one minute again and continue with one minute until you've had seven in a row. Then you can increase to three. For mindful eating to take hold you will need a regular meditation practice. Research on MB-EAT tells us that the more a person meditates the better his or her results. So, go for three minutes. I think you'll like it. Let's also go for three mindful bites each day. They can be the same food or different ones. Your choice.

***Today:* Eat three bites of food mindfully and meditate for three minutes.**

Today's Journal Question: **What are your thoughts about meditating so far?**

JANUARY 12:
BECOMING MINDFUL IN THE MOMENT

This journey is about mindful eating but becoming mindful in the everyday moments of your life will help your mindful eating and enhance your life. What do I mean by "mindful in the moment"? Simple. Right now, answer this question—where is your mind? You might be saying "reading this book, silly," but is it really? Your eyes may be on the page but is your mind there too? It is easy to wander off without even knowing or to go through the motions without really being present. I know I am not really reading the book in front of me when a few paragraphs go by and I can't remember what I read.

In those moments my eyes were on the page but my mind was elsewhere. There is nothing wrong with your mind going elsewhere. Simply notice where it's gone. I notice when I am watching TV, I sometimes miss some dialogue. Thank goodness for DVRs so I can rewind and relisten. Each time I do that I am refocusing my attention on what I am watching. Want to know something? My mind was elsewhere as I wrote this passage. While my fingers were busy typing on the keyboard my mind was imagining you reading this book. Minds wander. Mindfulness is simply noticing when they do.

For today, take a few moments throughout the day to notice where you mind is. Journal what you uncover. A simple trick to help you do this is to set your phone alarm to go off every few hours so you can check in.

Today: **Check in with your mind throughout the day to see where its focus is. Continue to eat three bites of food mindfully and meditate for three minutes.**

Today's Journal Question: **Reflect upon how being more mindful in your everyday life could help with your eating habits.**

JANUARY 13:
MINDFUL MOTHER NATURE . . .

One of the joys of becoming mindful is discovering how much more life has to offer. It's a way of noticing more of what has always been around you but that you may have never really paid much attention to. For example, how many trees surround your home? Even if you live in a city, there will be a tree somewhere. Where? What kind? Have you even noticed? When we are on a vacation, we tend to pay more attention to what is around us. Sometimes that's because the surroundings are new, so they seem more interesting. Other times it's maybe because we are more relaxed, so we are more open to what is happening around us.

We are surrounded by so much beauty every day that we take for granted or simply ignore. Spend a few minutes outside today noticing what is there. Pay attention to whatever gifts nature has bestowed to your little corner of the world. Look up to the sky and see the clouds. If it's raining, feel the wetness on your skin. If there is a flower, smell it. If a squirrel crosses your path follow it with your eyes. Live, if only for a moment, relishing the old adage "stop and smell the roses." For that moment life will really be sweet.

***Today:* Spend some time outdoors and observe Mother Nature. Continue eating your three mindful bites and meditating for three minutes.**

***Today's Journal Question:* What is your relationship with nature?**

JANUARY 14:
NEW AND IMPROVED?

If you are like I was you are in the habit of eating the same foods over and over again. You may have a few go-to breakfasts. Some favorite lunches and dinner entrées. You probably have some must-have snacks, too. The problem with having the same foods all the time is that such a routine can lead to mindless eating. You eat because it is there or allowed or easy. Becoming a mindful eater means really paying attention to your food choices and learning to enjoy a wide variety of tasty, satisfying and nutritious foods.

For today I would like you to go to the market and buy an item of food that you have never had before and think you may like. It can be a new piece of fruit or type of vegetable. It can be a prepared meal or fancy snack. Take the food item to a location where you can eat uninterrupted. That can be at home. In a park. Even in your car. If possible, eat the food when you are a little bit hungry (or at the very least not after you have had a full meal or snack). My reason for this suggestion will be explained at another time, but for now, try to be a little bit hungry.

When you are settled in the location where you will eat, take a moment to get centered. Adjust your seating so you are comfortable. Turn off all electronics. Take a few deep breaths. And when you are ready, turn your attention to your food and do the following:

- Put a bite of food on a fork, spoon or between your fingers.
- Look at it. Notice its colors and textures.
- Bring it to your nose and sniff. Notice its scent.
- Touch it to your lips. Feel its texture.
- Place it in your mouth, but don't chew. Feel it. Roll it over your tongue.
- Bite into it. Notice its flavor.
- Chew it slowly, savoring the flavor.
- When you are ready, swallow.
- Eat your food one bite at a time savoring each bite.
- Stop when you've had enough, or it stops tasting good, or it's gone.

When you are finished ask yourself if this is a food you might like to add to your repertoire of food choices. If yes, why yes? If no, why not? Try to do this exercise once a week to help you explore new foods and build your mindful eating skills.

***Today:* Go to the market and get a new food. Eat it mindfully as instructed above. Also, beginning today, eat one bite of every food you eat mindfully and continue to meditate for three minutes.**

***Today's Journal Question:* What would it be like for you to add new foods and beverages to your food repertoire?**

JANUARY 15:

OM . . .

The foundation for mindful eating is a daily mindfulness meditation practice. About ten days ago you began a one-minute meditation practice. Then we expanded it to three minutes. The purpose of that was to get you into the habit of meditating daily. Now we will expand your practice again to five minutes. You can use a guided meditation recording from an app or a CD.

The instructions for your expanded daily meditation practice are the same as for the shorter practice. To begin, simply:

- Find a comfortable place to sit or lie down.
- Loosen any tight-fitting clothing or shoes.
- Close your eyes.
- Take a deep breath in through your nose and then exhale through your mouth.
- Focus your attention on your breath and follow the guidance on the meditation recording.
- When your mind wanders, and it will, simply notice that is has done so and turn your attention back to your breath.
- When the recording is over, open your eyes and go back to your day.

If you don't want to use a guided meditation, you can set a timer for five minutes and go on your own. Do whatever serves you best. Try different guided meditations if you like. Make this practice your own. Set a goal of meditating at least six times during the week and keep track of your meditation practice in your journal.

***Today:* Eat one bite of each food you eat today mindfully and meditate for five minutes.**

***Today's Journal Question:* How does it feel to increase your meditation time to five minutes?**

JANUARY 16:
HOW DO I DO THIS MEDITATION THING?

Now that you are expanding your meditation practice to five minutes a day, it's time for some basic instructions on how to build a strong foundation for your practice. Starting off "right" will help you ease into a consistent practice without much extra effort. Here's how to start:

1. Choose a time which you can consistently set aside for your practice. Mornings, late afternoons, or early evenings are preferable to right before bed to prevent falling asleep.
2. Choose a special spot for your practice. Make it a sacred space that is used only for your practice and nothing else.
3. Choose your preferred posture—sitting, kneeling, or lying down. If you are not sure, start by sitting in a chair where you can main-

tain a relaxed but straight back. Some people like to sit cross-legged on a raised pillow. If you want to lie down, that's find just be sure not to get drowsy or you may fall asleep.

4. Choose the amount of time you will be practicing and set a timer (or use a timed guided meditation). If there are other people present when you are ready to practice, ask them not to disturb you. That includes pets and children!
5. If you like you can use headphones if you are listening to a guided meditation or to block out extraneous noise.
6. Now, begin your meditation. Please remember that learning to meditate is a skill and it may take a while for you to feel comfortable. If you notice you are judging yourself—"I'm too distracted." "I can't stop thinking." "This is too hard." "I'm too restless," etc.—simply observe these judgments as thoughts and return your attention back to your breath. In time, you will notice this will become easier. That is part of the practice.

Today: **Eat one bite of each food you eat today mindfully and meditate for five minutes.**

Today's Journal Question: **What do you think of meditating as a daily practice?**

JANUARY 17:
GOLDILOCKS AND A LESSON IN MINDFUL EATING

Once upon a time, in a far-off land, there lived a little girl named Goldilocks. One day, Goldilocks took a walk in the forest and came upon a house. She knocked on the door. No one answered so she walked in. Goldilocks saw three bowls of porridge sitting on the kitchen table. Hungry from her walk, she reached for the first bowl.

"This porridge is too hot!" she exclaimed and put the bowl down.

She reached for the second one. "This one is too cold," she noted disappointedly.

She tasted the porridge from the last bowl and said, "Oh, this porridge is exactly right," and then happily enjoyed her meal.

Little did you know when you heard the classic childhood story "Goldilocks and The Three Bears" that you were getting your first lesson in mindful eating. Goldilocks didn't eat the first bowl just because it was there.

Nor did she eat the second one because it was there. No, instead, she searched to find exactly the right one and then savored her meal.

How often do you eat something that is too hot or too cold or just not right because it is in front of you? How much more would you enjoy a meal or snack if it was "exactly right"? As you go about your day today, pay attention to if your food choices are "exactly right." If they are, great dig in. If they aren't, what can you do to choose differently?

Today: **Eat one bite of each food you eat today mindfully and meditate for five minutes.**

Today's Journal Question: **How does it feel to make sure that the food you eat is "just right" rather than simply accepting what is offered?**

JANUARY 18:

ANOTHER MINDFUL LESSON FROM OUR HEROINE GOLDILOCKS

Let's return to our heroine Goldilocks for another lesson in mindfulness. After Goldilocks mindfully ate the porridge, she felt sleepy, so she searched for some place to rest and found three beds.

She lay on the first and said, "This bed is too hard."

She lay on the second and said, "This bed is too soft."

When she lay down on the third bed she said, "This one is just right," and promptly fell asleep. Finding a comfortable position is as important to your meditation practice as finding a comfortable bed was for Goldilocks' sleep.

Some people like to sit on a chair. Others prefer a cushion. As for cushions, there are round ones, oval ones, square ones, flat ones, firm ones and ones that fold. If a cushion doesn't suit you, try a bench. There are specifically designed meditation benches that position you in such a way that you can meditate for a long time. You can also meditate on a bed or on the floor. Not sure how to decide? Google meditation cushions and you will find many websites to explore. Try out several options to find what works best for you. You may also find that what works best changes from time to time, even day to day. No worries. Just find a position where you will be comfortable and settle in.

Today: **Eat one bite of each food you eat today mindfully and meditate for five minutes.**

Today's Journal Question: **What will you do to find the right position for your meditation practice?**

JANUARY 19:

JUST BECAUSE IT'S LUNCH TIME DOESN'T MEAN YOU HAVE TO EAT

One of the skills you will develop as you become a mindful eater is learning to identify when you are truly hungry and when you want to eat just because it's meal time. We have been conditioned to eat three meals a day at specific times. As a result, we think we need to eat when mealtimes arrive. As it turns out you don't have to eat just because it's lunchtime. In fact, you will do your body a favor if you don't. What kind of favor you may be asking? Simple—digestion takes a lot of energy. If you eat when you are not hungry you will be adding food to your body's digestive load. Instead give it a rest. Notice if doing so gives you more energy, more ability to concentrate and more focus.

So, what do you do if it's lunchtime and you are not hungry for lunch? You have a few options. You can eat lunch mindfully knowing that you are not in fact hungry but are choosing to eat anyway. Or you can skip lunch and eat later when you are hungry. If this time is the only time you feel you will have to eat until much later and are concerned that you might get hungry at an inopportune time, have a small snack now. Eat your snack mindfully to buy yourself some time before your hunger returns. Over time, as you learn how best to feed your body, you may find yourself eating less food earlier in the day so that you are actually hungry at lunch time. The next time the clock strikes twelve ask yourself, "Am I really hungry or do I just want to eat because it's lunchtime?" and then make the mindful choice.

Today: **Eat one bite of each food you eat today mindfully and meditate for five minutes.**

Today's Journal Question: **How in touch are you with your hunger?**

JANUARY 20:

IF A CHERRY FALLS OFF A TREE, DOES IT MAKE A SOUND?

Have you ever listened to your food? Remember "snap, crackle and pop" of Rice Krispies fame? An important part of mindful eating is using all your senses to experience your food in the present moment. And hearing is a sense. So, listen to your food. The crackle of chopped onion as you drop it into a pan of hot oil, or the sound of sizzling fajitas. How about the sounds associated with preparing that food? The pop as you open a new jar of tomato sauce. The knife hitting the cutting board as you dice celery. The splash of water pouring from the faucet as you fill a pot to make pasta. The clank of a plate as you lay it on the table. Or the sounds in the deli as you and others order lunch. Our lives are filled with sound and yet so much of it goes unheard. Take a moment today to hear your food. Notice the sounds around you as you sit down for a meal. Get centered and listen to the melodiousness of sounds present.

Today: **Eat one bite of each food you eat today mindfully and meditate for five minutes.**

Today's Journal Question: **How tuned in are you to the sounds around you?**

JANUARY 21:

STAYING PRESENT IS A GIFT

Using your body is an excellent way to remember to stay present. For example, what is your posture like right now as you read this? If you are like me, you are slouching. I say this because as I am writing this I am slouching. Now that I am putting my attention on my posture, I can feel the roundedness of my shoulders and the pull in my lower back. Being aware, I choose to shift. I sit up straighter. I stretch my shoulders and relieve the pressure on my lower back. A moment of mindfulness and I feel physically better. What about you? What sensations are you observing at this moment? Mentally move through your body from head to toe and notice where you feel stiff, achy, or strong. Now stand up. Gently sway your body side to side. How does that feel? Where do you feel it? This is a very simple way of getting present. Practice bringing your attention to your body throughout the day. Do not underestimate the power that feeling your body gives you. Your mind and body will thank you.

Today: **Eat one bite of each food you eat today mindfully and meditate for five minutes.**

Today's Journal Question: **How can you use your body to stay present?**

JANUARY 22:

MAKING THE CUT

Mindful eating takes into account your own body's wisdom of what serves its needs best, as well as, guidance from nutritional science experts. We know from nutritional science that if your body takes in more food than it needs, it converts the excess food into fat, storing it for leaner times. In our overfed world, it is unlikely that leaner times will ever come so the excess fat our body is storing for us becomes the excess weight we carry around. When you get good at eating mindfully and eat per your body's instructions it is unlikely you will consume more food than you need. As you are learning these skills and getting better acquainted with your body's requirements, you can help yourself out by considering where you could cut down (even out) excess food without feeling deprived or hungry. For example, could you order a medium size beverage instead of a large? Could you share an order of fries with a friend? Could you put mayo on only one half of your sandwich? For the next few days, notice where it might be possible for you to cut down (or even out) your food intake. You don't have to do it, just notice how it might work if you did. By the way, today we up your meditation practice to eight minutes. Congratulations!

Today: **Eat one bite of each food you eat today mindfully and meditate for eight minutes.**

Today's Journal Question: **When could you choose a smaller portion and not feel deprived?**

JANUARY 23:

A MINDFUL CUP OF COFFEE

If you are like most Americans, your day starts off with a mug filled with scalding hot coffee which you gulp down as you rush to work by train, plane or automobile. Not a mindful way to begin the day, wouldn't you agree?

What if, just for today, you sipped your coffee as if you were in a Parisian café? What if, just for today, you savored your coffee? Really tasting each drop. Now maybe you can't do that with your morning cup of joe because you need to get to the office. But you probably could during one of your coffee breaks. Today, during one of those coffee breaks, make it a point to sit down and do nothing else but drink your coffee. Pay attention when you pour the coffee from the pot. Notice the pot. Is it heavy? Is it full? Is the coffee fresh or stale? Watch as the coffee fills your cup. Notice its aroma, its color. If you add cream, gently swirl it in and observe how the color and texture of the coffee changes. If you add sweetener, how much? Does the coffee need it? Why? What is your preference?

Now take the cup to your seat. Sit. Bring the cup to your lips and take a sip. Let the coffee linger on your tongue. Savor it. Is it to your liking? Does it need more cream or sugar? Is this a good cup of coffee or typical office swill? If it isn't good, why are you drinking it? If it tastes good, enjoy it. Sip it slowly with intention. Enjoy these few minutes alone with your brew. If it doesn't taste good, fix it. If you can't fix it, toss it. If you don't want to toss it think about what you could do differently to have a more delicious cup of coffee next time. Savoring a cup of coffee is practicing mindfulness. Making the coffee exactly as you like it is mindful too.

***Today:* Eat one bite of each food you eat today mindfully and meditate for eight minutes.**

***Today's Journal Question:* What would it be like to savor your coffee (or another beverage) today?**

JANUARY 24:
EVERYDAY MINDLESSNESS

We live on autopilot. This is not necessarily a bad thing. The idea that we do many things without having to think about them is good. For example, we breathe without having to remind our lungs to do their job. We walk and run without deliberately moving our legs. We do our morning routine (showering, brushing our teeth, and getting dressed) without much effort. These forms of "mindlessness"—doing without conscious thought or intention—help us. It's when we act mindlessly in other ways that we lose out. We live so much of our lives trying to get somewhere other than where we are. At work we pine for the weekend. In traffic we wish we were at work. When we are young, we want to be old. When we are old we want to be young. Here's the problem: When we want to be anywhere but where we are, we lose the gift of being present. Time passes and we are often filled we regret. When we are mindful, we are present. When we are mindless, we are not and when we are not, we miss so much. Our bodies are present but our minds are not. How many off-ramps have you missed in your life because we are daydreaming while driving? How many cookies did you eat before you reached the end of the tin? Most of the time our minds are not in the present. Our minds spend most of their time in the past, the future or fantasy. If this is true for you, don't feel bad. Join the club. Welcome to the human race! The good news is that you can change how mindless you are. Throughout the day check in with yourself and observe whether you are being mindless or mindful in that moment. You can set a reminder on your phone for the top of each hour as a way to do this. Then at the end of the day reflect on those moments when you found yourself being most mindful and when you were most mindless. Did any of those moments involve food?

Today: **Eat one bite of each food you eat today mindfully and meditate for eight minutes.**

Today's Journal Question: **What can you do to help yourself remember to be mindful throughout the day?**

JANUARY 25:
STOP, YOU MOVE TOO FAST, GOTTA MAKE THE MORNING LAST

Do you remember the old Paul Simon song "Feeling Groovy"? In it, Mr. Simon admonished all of us to slow down. Mindful eating makes the same request. A habit that many of us engage in is eating too fast. Often when we eat quickly, we miss the flavor, texture and satisfaction that the food offers. Rapid eating is often called mindless eating because we are eating without paying attention. We are not thinking about what we are doing, we just eat. For today, stop. Take a breath and eat a meal or snack more slowly. Allow yourself to really taste the food. Savor it. Take delight in it. Notice if doing so makes a difference in the amount food you eat throughout the day. I had an experience once when I chose to eat my dinner in this fashion. I deliberately sat down at my dining room table. Turned off the TV. Moved the phone. Got centered and ate my meal. I put my fork down between each bite and noticed the taste. I had prepared chicken tenders with steamed zucchini and some leftover mac and cheese.

By eating slowly and with intention I noticed a few things. I didn't really like the way I seasoned the chicken. Too strong. The zucchini was over steamed so it was a bit soggy. The mac and cheese was okay but not great. WOW! I know I am not a really good cook, but seriously! On any other day I would have eaten what was on my plate without paying attention and then reached for something sweet to end the meal. After really tasting the meal this time, I felt full and afterwards didn't need something sweet. What I need are cooking lessons! More on that later. . . Now it's your turn. Slow down once today and see what happens.

***Today:* Eat one bite of each food you eat today mindfully and meditate for eight minutes.**

***Today's Journal Question:* How might slowing down help you with your weight management goals?**

JANUARY 26:

LIVING IS HARD, EATING IS EASY

Life can be tough. We have good days. We have bad days. Sometimes it feels as if all we have are challenges, disappointments, setbacks, and loss. What do we do when times are rough? Where do we find relief? An escape? A break? For many of us, myself included, food is our solace. Eating is the behavior we choose to help us get through the uncomfortable times. In my previous books, I talked about getting through law school on peanut M&M's (yes, I was a lawyer before becoming a psychologist—but that is a story for another day). I joked that I wanted to write the Mars Company a thank you letter after earning my degree because if it weren't for their candy, I might not have gotten it! M&M's were my go-to stress releasers. And I wasn't the only one. During the last final exam of my first year, I noticed that the classmate sitting behind me had a gigantic bag of peanut M&M's sitting on his desk. Personally, I could not eat while taking a test but apparently, he could. When the exam ended and the professor called for us to hand it our papers, I turned to collect his and noticed the entire bag was empty. I understood. Food is comfort. Food helps us cope. Food is easy. When we eat to deal with our feelings (whether stress, sadness, anger or the like), we are emotionally eating. And emotional eating can be a big source of excess calories and excess weight.

Fortunately, mindfulness provides another way to cope with our emotional pain. Studies show us that mindfulness meditation is helpful in reducing stress and anxiety. A body scan meditation, for example, can relieve tension. So, the next time you want to eat in response to a problem, try a few minutes of mindful meditation first. If you still need to eat when you're done, eat. Chances are you won't need to or if you do, you'll eat less.

Today: **Eat one bite of each food you eat today mindfully and meditate for eight minutes.**

Today's Journal Question: **What role has emotional eating played in your weight loss struggle?**

JANUARY 27:
THE BEST DIET BEGINS WITH MINDFULNESS

Several years ago, I wrote a book called *The Best Diet Begins in Your Mind*. It is great little book designed to help people end emotional eating. It focuses on eight emotions and gives the reader practical tools for dealing with them. A premise of the book is that without dealing with one's emotions, every diet is doomed to fail. But if you address your emotions while you are dieting, any healthy diet can lead to successful weight loss. In other words, learning to manage your weight is as much about learning to manage your emotions as it is about managing your food. The book helps many people and I am proud of it.

It was after its publication, however, that I began studying mindfulness and mindful eating in depth. I have since learned the enormous value of mindfulness in handling emotions. Learning to be present with your emotions, becoming curious about them rather than afraid of them and no longer needing to eliminate them, can lead to a reduction in emotional eating in much the same way that applying practical tools can. Now I want to say that the best diet begins not only in your mind but also with mindfulness.

Applying mindfulness to your food choices and eating habits as well as to your emotional life is the most effective way I know to achieve permanent weight loss.

To be mindful of your emotions is to recognize them. One way to do that is to keep a feeling journal. Use your journal to observe your emotions, to become curious about them. How do they feel? Where in your body do you feel them? What triggered them? Is there a color associated with them?

How long do they last? Do they change in intensity or duration?

Emotions are part of being human. When you can embrace them rather than run from them you experience more of what being human is all about, and that's a good thing.

Today: **Eat one bite of each food you eat today mindfully and meditate for eight minutes.**

Today's Journal Question: **Choose one emotion you feel today and describe it as vividly as you can.**

JANUARY 28:
WHEN LESS IS MORE

One way to incorporate mindful eating into your daily routine is to identify ways in which you might start to eat healthier without giving up your favorite foods or feeling deprived. This is where utilizing reliable, scientifically supported nutritional advice comes into play. I call this cultivating Outer Guidance. We will work with Outer Guidance as we move along. One way to incorporate Outer Guidance is to be mindful of the nutritional value of the food you choose. The truth is nutrition matters. Now please keep in mind that mindful eating is a non-diet approach to weight management, so cultivating Outer Guidance is not about diet rules or restrictions. Instead, it is about being smart about your choices and choosing differently when possible.

Here's an example from my life. I love Starbucks' café mochas. Can't help it, I'm hooked. What I discovered as I embraced mindful eating is that I can enjoy a small size mocha as much as I enjoy a large size. I also noticed that a mocha made with non-fat milk tasted just as good to me as one made with 2% milk so I made that switch as well. By simply choosing to order the small non-fat version, I cut down on fat and calories without feeling deprived. This allows me to still enjoy my treat and manage my weight at the same time. Take some time today to think about one food or beverage which you can change. You don't have to change anything just start thinking about it. Where can you make less, more?

Today: **Eat one bite of each food you eat today mindfully and meditate for eight minutes.**

Today's Journal Question: **What food or beverage could you make a change**

to that would still allow you to enjoy it and also help you reach your weight management goals?

JANUARY 29:

YOUR BODY KNOWS BEST

Understanding your body's needs and how best to meet them is a core concept of mindful eating. If you are out of touch with your body, you may not know what is best for it. What I mean is that so much of what we eat and how much we eat is dictated by sources outside ourselves. For instance, if you are following a structured diet complete with food plan then you are eating according to its schedule which may or may not be your body's schedule. Or you dine out a lot and the amount of food you eat is based on the serving size provided. Or you grab a bag of this and a box of that and the amount contained in them is what you eat.

When you practice mindful eating, you tune into how much food your body needs when it needs it, which may or may not be consistent with the bag, box, restaurant, or meal plan serving. Beginning today, start paying attention to the serving sizes that show up. Ask yourself whether what is presented is the right amount for you or if you need more or less. If you need more, you can choose to have more. If you need less, you can choose to have less.

Today: **Eat one bite of each food you eat today mindfully and meditate for eight minutes.**

Today's Journal Question: **How will paying attention to serving sizes help you become a mindful eater?**

JANUARY 30:

HOW'S THE . . .OM. . . GOING FOR YOU?

If you have been traveling the journey I am setting out for you here, you have been practicing eight minutes of daily meditation—most days. If not, that's okay too. One of the principles of mindfulness is non-judgment. So, no judgment here. What we will do now is take some time to reflect on your experience so far. Here are some questions for you to consider:

1. Have I been consistent with my practice? If yes, how so? If not, what is getting in the way?
2. Have I found a posture that is comfortable for me? What works? What can I try out?
3. Have there been any changes to my eating habits? What changes am I noticing?
4. Have there been any improvements to my sleeping habits or energy levels? If so, what kind of improvements?
5. Can I focus more? Concentrate better?
6. Am I more motivated?
7. Is my life feeling more joyful?
8. Am I enjoying meditation? Why or why not?

As you move forward, continue meditating at least six times during the week with a goal towards having a daily practice.

***Today:* Eat one bite of each food you eat today mindfully and meditate for eight minutes.**

***Today's Journal Question:* How is your meditation practice going?**

JANUARY 31:
THINGS ARE AS THEY ARE

Equanimity is a great Scrabble word. It is also a great state of mind. Equanimity means calmness, composure, and levelheadedness. In a world filled with stress, uncertainty and pain, learning to cultivate equanimity is very helpful. You can use your meditation practice as a tool to develop it by choosing to focus your attention on the following thoughts: "Things are as they are. May I accept things as they are." Repeating these phrases to yourself can still a worried mind. When you calm your mind, you reduce the need to eat to soothe yourself, and it is easier to eat mindfully when you have a peaceful mind.

***Today:* Eat one bite of each food you eat today mindfully and meditate for eight minutes.**

***Today's Journal Question:* How can learning to cultivate equanimity help you?**

February

FEBRUARY 1:

WHAT'S HUNGER GOT TO DO WITH IT?

Back in 1984 Tina Turner's song "What's Love Got to Do with It" gained worldwide acclaim. Her lyrics questioned whether love has anything to do with physical attraction. We can ask the same question about hunger and eating. Does hunger have anything to do with eating? In the world of mindful eating the answer is a resounding yes! One of the first skills of mindful eating is learning to understand your body's hunger language. How do you know when it is time to eat? Can you tell when you are physically hungry? Or, do you eat according to the clock or because food is available?

In a world where food is everywhere and we don't know the meaning of true hunger, this question may seem odd. But it is an important one. Pay attention to how your body signals that it needs food. Do you get a stomach pang? A headache? Dizzy? When your body needs food, it tells you. Listen. If you feed it when it is hungry and don't when it's not, you will go a long way to meeting your weight loss goal. Check in with your body before each meal or snack to see if you are feeling hungry. Start becoming familiar with how this element of Inner Wisdom works for you. Also, it's time to add two minutes to your meditation practice—Woohoo!

***Today:* Eat one bite of each food you eat today mindfully and meditate for ten minutes.**

***Today's Journal Question:* How does your body let you know that you are hungry?**

FEBRUARY 2:

MINI-MEDITATIONS—THE EASY WAY TO MINDFUL EATING

An easy and effective way to get yourself to pay more attention to what you are eating is to do a mini-meditation before your meal or snack. A mini-meditation simply means pausing, taking a few deep breaths, letting go of any tension, and becoming aware of the food you are about to eat. Practice a mini-meditation once a day, either before a snack or meal, to build your mindful eating skills. Here's how to do it:

- Begin by taking two or three deep breaths, letting the air flow all the way into your stomach, and then flow gently back out again
- Close your eyes and let your breathing find its own natural, comfortable rhythm and depth, and gently focus your attention on the feeling of your breath as it comes in at the tip of your nose, moves through the back of your throat, into your lower diaphragm, and back out again, letting your stomach rise and fall naturally with each breath
- Release any tension you may be feeling
- If you notice any thoughts, emotions or feelings that arise, simply bring your awareness back to your breath
- Now we are going to bring your attention to the experience of eating
- Picture the food in front of you
- Without judgment, notice any feelings, experiences, or thoughts that are going through your mind, particularly any related to choosing to eat at this moment or related to the food in front of you
- Release any tension you may be feeling
- Now make the choice to eat the food in front of you with mindful enjoyment
- Take one more deep breath and when you are ready, open your eyes

Today: **Do a mini-meditation before one meal or snack and meditate for ten minutes.**

Today's Journal Question: **How does it feel to pause and do a mini-meditation before you eat?**

FEBRUARY 3:

INTENTIONAL MINDFUL EATING

Beginning today, intentionally eat one meal or snack each day mindfully. This means choosing your foods deliberately, starting with a mini-meditation, applying techniques from the raisin experience and paying attention to your physical hunger. It does NOT necessarily mean eating all your food very slowly! Simply get into the mindset of mindful eating and enjoy your meal or snack in a mindful way. Record in your journal what this experience felt like. Notice what effect eating this way has on your mood, your food choices the rest of the day, and how the experience may vary from day to day.

Today: Do a mini-meditation before one meal or snack, eat one meal or snack mindfully and meditate for ten minutes.

Today's Journal Question: **How is mindful eating is different than your normal way of eating?**

FEBRUARY 4:

SHHH? YOU CAN'T SILENCE THE CHATTERING MIND

Have you noticed that your mind is busy twenty-four hours a day every day? Thoughts, conversations, to-do lists, arguments, plans, regrets, you name it, fill our minds all the time. In the meditation world, we call this the "Chattering Mind." As you establish your meditation practice you may become even more aware of this chatter than ever before. This awareness may make it feel as if meditation is impossible. What is impossible is trying to quiet the jabbering. Your objective in your meditation practice is not to silence these pesky thoughts but rather to become aware of them. Noticing them without judgment. Becoming curious about your mind, how it works and the thoughts that occupy it.

If your chattering mind is too distracting and you feel as if you cannot meditate, don't give up. Instead count your breaths. Counting your breaths is a way to focus your attention away from the relentless noise in your head and calm the mind. You can count your breaths by assigning a number to each in-breath starting with one and counting up to ten. When you reach ten begin again with one. If you don't reach ten, in other words, your mind wanders, start over with one as soon as you realize that you've lost count. You can count like this for a minute or two or for however long feels right to you.

Today: **Do a mini-meditation before one meal or snack, eat one meal or snack mindfully and meditate for ten minutes.**

Today's Journal Question: **What does your "Chattering Mind" have to say?**

FEBRUARY 5:
THANK THE GROCER

One step in the mindful eating process is acknowledging and expressing gratitude to all who participated in bringing you the food you eat. From the farmers who harvested the produce to the manufacturer who put it in a box to the grocers who stocked the shelves, each played a role in the meal you are about to eat. Unless you live on a farm it is unlikely that you give this idea much thought. We city folk take much of what we eat for granted. Being mindful means paying attention to the process of growing, preparing and delivering our food. When I began eating mindfully, I also began cooking more. Before then, I relied a lot on prepared foods. I used to call Whole Foods my personal chef because every week I would stock on their prepared salads, sandwiches and entrées. There is nothing wrong with using prepared foods but for me as I adopted mindful eating I wanted to cook more.

My favorite time to shop is Sunday mornings around 7am. The reason I like that time is that the store is empty and the aisles are filled with clerks busy restocking the shelves and bins. I use this time to ask for help—help choosing a ripe melon, help deciding between different cuts of meat, help picking wild-caught seafood. With so few customers around, the staff is available and eager to help. I am grateful to these men and women for their knowledge and assistance, and I let them know. So, the next time you are in the grocery store, thank the produce guy, the stock clerk, and the cashier for the help they are giving you in getting scrumptious food on your table.

Today: **Do a mini-meditation before one meal or snack, eat one meal or snack mindfully and meditate for ten minutes.**

Today's Journal Question: **For whom can you feel grateful today?**

FEBRUARY 6:
THE DELICIOUS TOOTSIE ROLL CENTER

One of my favorite candies is a Tootsie Roll lollipop. I especially like the chocolate-flavored ones, although the purple ones are good too. Here's the problem I have with these luscious treats. I bite into them! I don't start out that way but quickly I become impatient and go straight for the chewy center. As an experiment, I tried to eat one of the lollipops mindfully. Here's what I did.

I purchased a package of lollipops and brought them home. I placed the bag on my table and sat down. There was nothing else on the table but the bag of pops. I began my mindful eating with the bag. First, I silently thanked the Tootsie Roll Company for making the pops. Then I thanked the grocery store where I purchased it from and all the people I could think of who had a hand in getting the bag to me. Then I picked the bag up, feeling its weight in my hands. I tossed it gently from side to side. I admired its colors and graphics. When I was ready, I opened the bag. I poured all the pops onto the table and studied them. I carefully choose the one I wanted to eat and put the rest back in the bag. I set the bag aside. I held my chosen pop up in the air and took pleasure in my choice. I carefully unwrapped it, setting the wrapping aside. Now I gave the pop my full attention. I noticed its color and texture. I saw where it was bumpy and where it was smooth. I touched my lips with it and then drew in its scent.

Funny, it didn't smell as chocolatey as I expected it would. I placed the lollipop in my mouth and rolled it around. I let my tongue play with it a bit. I noticed the flavor starting to emerge. Delicious. Now for the hard part. I left the lollipop in my mouth without chewing it. I licked it. Sucked it. It took a long time to dissolve. I felt my impatience rising. I paid attention to the thoughts and feelings I was having. I felt the resistance to waiting. "This is taking forever. I can't do this. I want to take a bite!" But I waited and I refocused my attention away from my thoughts and back on the pop. Slowly, I savored the pop taking ten minutes to reach the center. There it was—the tempting, alluring chocolate center. Again, I noticed the urge to bite into it. I observed my thoughts and feelings. Some of which reflected pride in having come this far.

Once again, I turned my attention to the lollipop and let it dissolve slowly in my mouth. I surrendered to the experience and felt really good. When I got to the white stick I was done. I placed the stick inside the wrapper and sat for a moment. I thought back on what I had just done. I smacked my lips to taste the lingering flavor and I got up. I tossed the used wrapper into the trash and went on with my day feeling pleased and happy. I was proud of what I had done. Proud of the step I took towards mindful eating. And the lollipop was so satisfying I didn't crave sweets for the rest of the day.

Want to try this for yourself? Do you think you can mindfully eat a Tootsie Roll lollipop without biting or chewing? If these lollipops aren't your thing, find another candy treat and eat it mindfully.

***Today:* Do a mini-meditation before one meal or snack, eat one meal or snack mindfully and meditate for ten minutes.**

***Today's Journal Question:* What would it mean for you if you could eat treats mindfully?**

FEBRUARY 7:

PLAY WITH YOUR FOOD

There was a Chinese restaurant on Long Island, where I grew up, that was our family's favorite. Whenever we celebrated a special occasion, we would go there. My parents would treat themselves to a Pu-Pu Platter filled with a delicious assortment of Chinese appetizers while my sister and I sipped our "Shirley Temples." (In case you don't know what a "Shirley Temple" is, it is a non-alcoholic drink made up of ginger ale and maraschino cherries.) We loved those drinks but our favorite part was at the end of the meal making concoctions with what was left in our glass. We would put in tea, sugar, salt, pepper, rice, you name it. Whatever we could find. We would giggle at our creations while our parents rolled their eyes. I bring up the "Shirley Temples" to remind you of what fun playing with your food can be. Think of a two-year-old laughing as she tosses peas on the floor or mushing cake into her mouth at birthday time. While it may not be very "adult" to play with your food, for the purposes of mindful eating, please do.

I am not suggesting you throw your peas on the floor (although you can if you want to.) I am suggesting that you find ways to take delight in your food. For example, cut radishes into the shape of flowers before putting them in your salad. Serve your cereal in a crystal bowl. Fill your plate with foods from all colors of the rainbow. Use exotic spices. Try new recipes. Eat different cuisines. Mix and match flavors and textures. Eat outside your "box." Many of us are stuck in food ruts, habitually eating the same foods all the time. We do this for several reasons. One, it is convenient. Two, it is easy. Three, we are afraid that if we deviate, we will gain weight. Now that you are exploring mindful eating, try new foods. Be willing to try something unusual. Discover what else you like when you eat outside your box. You may be pleasantly surprised.

***Today:* Do a mini-meditation before one meal or snack, eat one meal or**

snack mindfully and meditate for ten minutes.

***Today's Journal Question:* What foods or cuisine could you sample that would be outside your box?**

FEBRUARY 8:

OLD MACDONALD HAD A FARM

If you have the good fortune to be living in a rural community you most likely have access to the freshest, most delicious food available. For the rest of us, living in the city or the suburbs we need to go in search of such treasures. Fortunately, most cities and towns now bring the fresh produce and products via farmer's markets and co-ops. If you have never been to a farmer's market you are missing out. Most farmer's markets have local vendors setting up stall after a stall of ripe, inviting produce and other freshly made products, such as bread, honey, and jam. The reason to go to these markets is to obtain the best food around. Trust me, the taste of a ripe tomato straight off the vine is so much better than anything you can find in a supermarket. Google "farmer's markets" in your neighborhood and make it a point to go to one this week. Walk around. Enjoy the samples. Bring home something delicious and then savor it. It's like heaven on earth.

***Today:* Do a mini-meditation before one meal or snack, eat one meal or snack mindfully and meditate for ten minutes.**

***Today's Journal Question:* Visit a Farmer's Market or Co-Op and afterwards reflect on how incorporating regular visits to such venues could enhance your mindful eating.**

FEBRUARY 9:

LESS OF A GOOD THING

There is a good chance that by now you are naturally eating less. If not, it is time to mindfully cut back. Mindfulness, unlike dieting, is not about deprivation. But that said, it is not about gluttony either. Some people, when they start eating mindfully, overindulge because they mistakenly think that not restricting means they can eat anything. You can eat anything you want—just not all at the same time! If you have been overdoing it, it's time to cut back. Think about when you can eat less without feeling deprived and try to cut back. Pay attention to how doing this makes you feel. If this is too difficult to do, try choosing a food or beverage that you feel neutral about (meaning you can take it or leave it) and cut back on that. Cutting back on favorites especially at the beginning can lead to a sense of loss, which may lead to overeating. Starting today, mindfully eat less of something you feel neutral about and see how that makes you feel. Hopefully, wonderful!

***Today:* Do a mini-meditation before one meal or snack, eat one meal or snack mindfully and meditate for ten minutes.**

***Today's Journal Question:* What is it like for you to mindfully eat less of something you feel neutral about?**

FEBRUARY 10:
EVERYDAY THANKS

My favorite holiday is Thanksgiving. One reason is that my birthday falls near Thanksgiving so there is always a lot of celebrating. Another reason is that I love the food served. I have wonderful memories of my father waking up at dawn to prepare the turkey. By the time I awoke the house was filled with the aroma of roasting bird. Years later when we celebrated Thanksgiving in my sister's home, he would still make the turkey and we would drive the hour to her place with the turkey on the backseat. Boy, did the inside of the car smell heavenly! My dad's turkey wasn't the only delicacy. Our table was teeming with scrumptious varieties of vegetables, potatoes, stuffing, and pies. If you celebrate a traditional American Thanksgiving, I am sure your table is the same. I bring up Thanksgiving now because giving thanks is an integral part of mindful eating. Just as we acknowledge how the food got to our plate, with mindful eating, we also give thanks for the food itself. We express gratitude for its presence, its nutrition, its taste. We show appreciation for the variety and abundance of food we have available to us. This appreciation can be part of the mindful eating experience. For example, you can say or think a thought of gratitude as you sit down to eat. Gratitude can also be felt when shopping for food. That's when I feel especially grateful. I stand in awe in the produce department mindful of all the choices I have. Just walking up and down the aisles of any typical American supermarket could evoke such feelings. We have so much available to us. How fortunate we are. Being mindful is being aware. When we are aware it is hard not to be grateful. Take a moment today to feel thankful for the food you eat today. Express your thankfulness in whatever way suits you best.

***Today:* Do a mini-meditation before one meal or snack, eat one meal or snack mindfully and meditate for ten minutes.**

***Today's Journal Question:* In your journal describe ten people, events, circumstances, or objects for which you feel grateful and why.**

FEBRUARY 11:

HARNESSING THE POWER OF THE SCALE FOR GOOD NOT EVIL

Back in January we discussed weighing yourself and the role of the scale. At that time, I asked you to not weigh yourself more than once a week. Today we will explore why in greater detail. By choosing to address your eating and food habits using the mindful approach, you are going to be measuring your success in ways that may be different than the ways you may have used in the past. Our focus is not going to be just on the number on the scale. Our focus is on how we use our Inner Wisdom and Outer Guidance, how we improve our state of mind, and how well we cope with our emotions without eating. Yes, it is true that research shows that those who are most successful at weight loss weigh themselves to get feedback, but too frequent weighing is counter-productive.

Weighing daily, for example, puts too much attention on the number on the scale in a way that is judgmental, rather than mindful. Weighing yourself once per week is often enough to get evidence of how your efforts are working. Weighing once a week (or even once a month) uses the number on the scale as information rather than an indictment of you. Learning to use the scale as a feedback tool rather than an assessment of your self-worth is a worthwhile endeavor and is consistent with what you are trying to accomplish by being a mindful eater—more self-acceptance and peace of mind. Think of the number on the scale as offering information about how your behaviors are impacting your weight. The number does not mean that you are "good" or "bad" but rather that you may need to do something differently if you are not seeing gradual weight loss.

***Today:* Do a mini-meditation before one meal or snack, eat one meal or snack mindfully and meditate for ten minutes.**

Today's Journal Question: **What role has your scale played in your previous attempts to lose weight?**

FEBRUARY 12:
STAY PUPPY STAY

One meditation teacher I had told me that "meditating is like training a young puppy to stay." Think about it. You place the puppy on a spot on the floor and tell it to stay. It may stay there for a moment or two but sooner rather than later it gets up and walks away. Since it does not know better, you don't scold it or yell at it. You simply pick it up, put it back where it was, and say "stay," perhaps rewarding it with a small treat or gentle pat. Soon it walks away again, and you return it to its spot. Gradually, it learns to stay for longer periods of time before it gets up. In time it learns the command "stay" and your efforts will have paid off. The same can be said about your thoughts. Your wandering mind is like the puppy. Your task is to return your mind to your breath each time it wanders off. Like training the puppy, training your mind to manage distracting thoughts and sensations while meditating is a process that develops slowly with practice. So, when you are meditating and your mind wanders, which it will, treat it like you would a sweet puppy and simply return it to its spot, which for you is your breath.

Today: **Do a mini-meditation before one meal or snack, eat one meal or snack mindfully and meditate for ten minutes.**

Today's Journal Question: **How is your mind like a puppy?**

FEBRUARY 13:
GOLD STARS AND STICKERS

I am all for rewards and reminders. For many years as a university professor, I would reward my college-aged students with stickers for reading their textbooks. I had stars, smiley faces, and "you did it" emblems among others. Even though most of the students hadn't gotten a sticker from a teacher since grade school, and might have thought they were childish, they expressed great delight is receiving them. You can, too, by placing a gold star or other sticker in your journal for jobs well-done. Whether you did your meditation practice or ate your lunch mindfully, reward yourself. Practice acknowledging yourself for the positive actions you take (or the harmful ones you don't take). See your progress in terms of small success rather than waiting for the big result—like a big weight loss.

If you are struggling to do take the actions you want to take to become a mindful eater, use stickers as reminders. Place stickers strategically around your kitchen or office to remind yourself to do the mini-meditations, take a breath before eating, to savor your food, etc. Such reminders can help you stay on track and reinforce your mindful eating habits.

***Today:* Do a mini-meditation before one meal or snack, eat one meal or snack mindfully and meditate for ten minutes.**

***Today's Journal Question:* What rewards and reminders can you use to help you with the new skills you are learning?**

FEBRUARY 14:
EAT WHAT YOU LOVE, LOVE WHAT YOU EAT

Happy Valentine's Day! Before you dive into that box of chocolates, let's get mindful! Today is a day that many associate with love. Here's a question for you—do you love the food you eat? By that I mean, do you choose to eat foods you really enjoy? Are you sure? Have you really tasted the foods you claim to enjoy? Let's consider that box of chocolates. Do you dive in, popping one chocolate into your mouth after another, or do savor each morsel? Do you taste what you are eating or do you take large bites and swallow quickly? When I started mindful eating, I noticed that foods that I thought I loved I really didn't love once I truly tasted them. Now, I reject those former favorites and choose, instead, new preferences. Eating food you love does not mean overeating them or eating them quickly. It means tasting and savoring the foods you choose. Practice choosing food you love. See if doing so results in a more satisfying eating experience.

***Today:* Do a mini-meditation before one meal or snack, eat one meal or snack mindfully and meditate for ten minutes.**

***Today's Journal Question:* Do you eat foods you love, why or why not?**

FEBRUARY 15:

REMIND ME—WHY AM I MEDITATING?

It's been about six weeks since you began this journey to mindful eating and a big part of your journey has been starting a meditation practice. At this point you may be wondering, why am I doing this again? To answer that question, let me review three reasons for using meditation as a tool for mindful eating.

- Meditation is a method to become more aware of automatic thoughts, feelings and behaviors. Since mindless and emotional eating are, for the most part, automatic, meditation gives a way to interrupt these habitual responses and create space for something different.
- Learning to be aware of the breath and quiet the "chattering mind" allows us to be more in the present, to identify what is going on right now and to choose how we want to think, feel, act and eat.
- By stopping automatic reactions and creating a pause, we bring a moment of relaxation into our otherwise hectic lives.

When you put these three reasons together you can see how they create the opportunity for a new and improved relationship with food and eating. If you are working on your daily practice, good for you. If you haven't started or are having trouble, no worries. You can always start again.

***Today:* Do a mini-meditation before one meal or snack, eat one meal or snack mindfully and meditate for ten minutes.**

***Today's Journal Question:* What reasons could compel you to start and maintain a meditation practice?**

FEBRUARY 16:

DOES LEFTOVER FOOD MAKE YOU ANXIOUS?

As you get better at mindful eating you may leave food on your plate. You will most likely feel satisfied with less food than you serve yourself so there will be leftovers. Is that okay? What does it feel like to leave food over? Do you feel guilty? Anxious? Proud? If you do have leftovers in the fridge, say a doggie bag from dinner last night, how does that feel? Does the doggie bag call your name? Is its presence in the fridge distracting for you? Do you think about it? Find it hard to concentrate knowing that it's there? If these questions sound familiar, you are in good company. Many people feel the same way.

Why do you feel this way? What does it mean to you to leave food over? Why is it hard? Do you feel deprived? Taking a mindful stance, simply notice, without judgment, what comes up for you when you leave food on your plate. With time, you will get good at serving yourself the right amount of food to meet your hunger levels so there will be less leftover. You will also get comfortable being in the presence of leftovers. Until then, observe what's going on and explore the reasons why.

Today: **Do a mini-meditation before one meal or snack, eat one meal or snack mindfully and meditate for ten minutes.**

Today's Journal Question: **What happens for you when you leave food on your plate?**

FEBRUARY 17:
GORILLAS IN THE MIDST

If you ever took a Psych 101 or Intro to Sociology class in high school or college, you may be familiar with the famous Gorilla on the Basketball Court study. To refresh your memory, students are asked to watch a video of a basketball game. They are asked to count the number of times the team in the white jerseys passed the ball to each other. While the players are passing the ball around, a man dressed as a gorilla walks onto the court. He stops in the middle of the court, beats his chest and then walks away. When the video ended, the students are asked to reveal their count. Then they are asked if anyone noticed the gorilla. The majority of them did not! They were so sure there was no gorilla they asked to watch the video again.

Much to their surprise, the gorilla was there. This study was to demonstrate something known as selective attention. Selective attention means that we tune out unimportant details and focus our attention on what really matters. In the case of the students, their attention was on basketball players so they missed the gorilla. One could say they were mindful of the basketball but mindless about the gorilla. How much do you miss in life because of where your attention is directed? When you are so focused on one event than you neglect the rest? If you eat while you are working on your computer or watching TV or driving while you eat, where is your attention? Are you paying full attention anywhere? If your attention is in one direction, what effect does that have on your other activities? For today, try to do one activity with full awareness. Give whatever task is in front of you—brushing your teeth, driving to school, preparing your lunch, eating your dinner—your full attention. If you do, what happens? How does it feel? Do you notice the gorilla in your midst?

***Today:* Do a mini-meditation before one meal or snack, eat one meal or snack mindfully and meditate for ten minutes.**

***Today's Journal Question:* Where might selective attention be playing a part in your life?**

FEBRUARY 18:

WHAT WILL PEOPLE THINK . . . ?

Overeating has become an American pastime. We eat all the time. At ballgames and concerts. At weddings and funerals. At the beach, the pool, the lake. While driving, while shopping. When we are on the phone or on the computer. We eat when we watch TV, read a book or go to the movies. I recently went to a movie theater that served a full café and bar menu at your seat. All this available food leads to overeating. So, what happens if you make the decision to stop? What happens if you make the decision to eat according to your body's needs and not whenever food is offered? I ask these questions to new mindful eaters and silence permeates the room. They become visibly uncomfortable and then start offering answers including: "I would feel left out." "People would judge me or criticism me." "I will be made fun of." "I'll feel different." "I don't know how to say no." "I'll draw unwanted attention to myself." "People will think I am on yet another diet and not take me seriously." I get it. Becoming a mindful eater makes you different.

People around you may get uncomfortable or not understand what you are doing. Changing your relationship to food can feel like an uphill battle. It can feel as if you are the only one trudging up the mountain and everybody else is at base camp partying and living it up. The truth is change can be hard. Change can subject us to ridicule from others who do not have the bravery to do as we are doing. It takes courage, self-compassion and patience to embrace mindful eating but the rewards are worth it. You don't have to convince anyone of this truth because it will show. Eventually people will want what you have. Then you can introduce them to mindful eating. Meanwhile, simply, politely refuse what is offered and turn your attention to another activity. That is mindfulness in action.

***Today:* Do a mini-meditation before one meal or snack, eat one meal or snack mindfully and meditate for ten minutes.**

***Today's Journal Question:* How can you address people's concerns, criticisms, and curiosity about mindful eating?**

FEBRUARY 19:

THE RIVER'S EDGE

Have you ever had the pleasure of sitting at a river's edge and watching the movement of the water? Can you imagine it? Can you see the ripples? How about tree branches and twigs drifting by? Our thoughts are like the ripples and objects in the river, floating by us without our interference. You can use the idea of a river to understand the nature of your mind. Our thoughts are like the water and items in the river. They flow into our awareness and, unless we grab onto them and hold on for dear life, glide right out again. Imagine a branch in the river. You see it. You can think about it—wondering where it came from, how long it's been there—or you can simply watch it as it sails out of sight. The lesson here is that you do not have to act on your thoughts, whether in your imagination or in real life. When you have a thought about food you can choose to just observe it. Watch it as it floats into your awareness and watch as it floats away. Imagine the food gliding atop the glistening river as it sails out of view.

***Today:* Do a mini-meditation before one meal or snack, eat one meal or snack mindfully and meditate for ten minutes.**

***Today's Journal Question:* What would happen if you were able to watch your thoughts sail by without reacting to them?**

FEBRUARY 20:

THE MORE YOU PRACTICE THE MORE YOU LOSE

The research on mindfulness-based eating awareness offers an incentive for developing and maintaining a meditation practice. A study published by Drs. Kristeller, Wolever and Sheets in 2011 showed a direct correlation between the amount of meditating a person does and an improvement in her ability to control her eating and in the amount of weight she lost. In other words, the more you do, the more you lose. Whenever you feel as if you don't want to meditate, remember these results and gently (and with compassion) encourage yourself to keep on keeping on.

***Today:* Do a mini-meditation before one meal or snack, eat one meal or snack mindfully and meditate for ten minutes.**

***Today's Journal Question:* If you haven't been able to create a daily practice yet, what is holding you back?**

FEBRUARY 21:
MINDSETS FOR MINDFUL EATING

The ultimate gift of taking a mindful eating approach to food is a shift in your relationship with food and eating. This shift will not happen overnight but it will happen over time. Overeating, binge eating, emotional eating, and making poor food choices are habits that have been around for a long time. Altering your mindset can assist in your journey and foster conditions for success.

Try these attitudes on for your new mindful eating mindset:

- Be curious and playful as you incorporate mindful eating into your life. Judgment and self-criticism will undermine your efforts. Release them.
- Focus on making small, incremental changes. Sweeping changes can be too anxiety producing and consequently defeat your intentions.
- Make changes that you will be able to continue for the indefinite future. We are making changes that you can continue for the rest of your life. This is not a temporary fix.
- Redefine the purpose of food in your life. Instead of using food as entertainment or medicine, look to food as a means for supporting life, for giving you the strength and energy you need to lead a meaningful and fulfilling life.

***Today:* Do a mini-meditation before one meal or snack, eat one meal or snack mindfully and meditate for ten minutes.**

Today's Journal Question: **Adopt one of these attitudes for the day and then reflect upon your experience in your journal.**

FEBRUARY 22:

EATING WITH INTENTION

Mindful Eating is sometimes defined as eating with awareness and intention. What does it mean to eat with intention? If we think of intention as being something you plan to do, how might that apply to eating? When we eat, we have many intentions. We have the intention to feed ourselves. We have the intention to eat a particular food or at a particular place. We have the intention to pick up the utensil or use our fingers to eat the food. We can also intend to eat for nourishment. To eat only when we are hungry and stop when we are full. To eat for satisfaction and satiety. To eat foods that taste good. To turn down food that does not serve us. How intentional are you about the food you eat and how you eat it? Does your intention change? If so, how does it change? What thoughts show up? What feelings are there? Before you have your next meal or snack, check in with yourself about your intentions and see if your actions reflect them.

Today: **Do a mini-meditation before one meal or snack, eat one meal or snack mindfully and meditate for ten minutes.**

Today's Journal Question: **What might improve if you practiced being intentional about your food and eating habits?**

FEBRUARY 23:

QUICK CHECK-IN

As Joey Tribbiani of *Friends* fame asks, "How you doin'?" take a moment and check in with yourself. How are you feeling physically? Any aches? Tingles? Numbness? Are you tired, full of energy? What about your mood? Are you happy? Sad? Angry? Flat? What are you thinking? Are you in the past? Present? Future? Check in with yourself periodically and notice, without judgment, what's going on. If you are focused on food, how fat you are, or how much you ate last night, no worries. Offer yourself compassion and understanding. Take a few breaths, center yourself and go on with your day.

Today: **Do a mini-meditation before one meal or snack, eat one meal or snack mindfully and meditate for ten minutes.**

Today's Journal Question: **How might checking in with yourself and figuring out "How you doin'" affect your relationship to food, your eating habits and yourself?**

FEBRUARY 24:

ARE YOU TUNED INTO HUNGER?

Earlier this month I asked you to start becoming aware of how your body lets you know you are hungry. Today we will dive deeper into this topic. The research on mindful eating tells us that people can learn to become aware of how hungry they are. While each of us may experience hunger differently, it is possible for you to learn what your unique hunger levels are. A tool used in MB-EAT is the Hunger Awareness Scale. With this scale you rate your hunger from one (not hungry) to ten (very hungry) before, during and after a meal or snack.

To create your own Hunger Awareness Scale, describe how you feel when you are not hungry at all (one). For example, you may feel whole, focused on other activities, content. Then figure out what moderately hungry feels like for you (five); for example, you notice some grumbling in your stomach and your concentration is off. Lastly, describe how you feel when you are very hungry (ten); for example, irritable, impatient, headachy. Looking at your descriptions, identify what level of hunger is the best level for you to eat something. For most people that level is between four and five. Eating when you are overly hunger can lead to excess eating so practice getting to know your hunger levels and eating at the right level for you.

As practice, eat one meal and one snack mindfully each day paying special attention to your level of physical hunger before, during and afterwards. See what patterns you notice and when you feel your best.

Today: **Do a mini-meditation before one meal or snack, eat one meal or snack mindfully and meditate for ten minutes.**

Today's Journal Question: **If you are open to creating a Hunger Awareness Scale for yourself, how will you use it? If not, why not?**

FEBRUARY 25:
WHAT AM I REALLY HUNGRY FOR?

Central to tuning into your physical hunger signals is learning how to distinguish them from other eating triggers, such as emotional, social or environmental ones. Inner Wisdom comes from understanding how you experience these eating triggers and acquiring the skills to respond accordingly. Today we will focus on emotional triggers. Emotional triggers can mimic physical signals. For example, you many feel nervousness in your stomach and confuse it for hunger. Emotional triggers are also associations you have made between feeling states and particular foods. Do you devour a bag of chips whenever you are angry? Is ice cream the food that soothes your hurt feelings?

Eating in response to emotions is commonplace. People call it eating to soothe or comfort eating. We all do. In and of itself it is not a terrible thing. It's when we do it all the time, to the exclusion of other ways of managing our emotions, that we get into trouble. Mindful eating teaches us to distinguish between true physical hunger which is our body's way of requesting nourishment and emotional hunger which is our mind's way of demanding relief. To help you differentiate between physical and emotional hunger, ask yourself, "What Am I Really Hungry for?" If the answer is a good cry, you won't find it in the fridge.

***Today:* Do a mini-meditation before one meal or snack, eat one meal or snack mindfully and meditate for ten minutes.**

***Today's Journal Question:* What are you really hungry for?**

FEBRUARY 26:
IT'S MY PARTY AND I'LL EAT IF I WANT TO

Another time when we may eat when we are not be physically hungry is when we are involved with social activities. Social cues to eat abound and if you are not mindful you may fall prey to them without even noticing. Are any of these situations familiar to you?

- You have popcorn every time you go to the movies.
- You can't see a ballgame without a hot dog or two.
- When you see your friends for coffee you always order something to eat.

- You overeat at Sunday family dinners.
- You keep pie in the house "just in case" someone drops by.
- Every time you see a particular relative, she insists on feeding you and you can't say no.

These are some typical examples of eating because we are in a social setting and not because we are physically hungry. Being mindful under these conditions means either choosing not to eat (because you are not hungry) or choosing to eat while being aware of your decision and allowing it to be without judgment or self-recrimination. The next time you are in social setting that offers food, observe your reactions and make a mindful decision on how to proceed. With mindfulness, you can't go wrong.

***Today:* Do a mini-meditation before one meal or snack, eat one meal or snack mindfully and meditate for ten minutes.**

***Today's Journal Question:* How do social activities affect your eating?**

FEBRUARY 27:

WHEN FOOD IS ENTERTAINMENT

Similar to eating in response to social cues is using food for entertainment. When there is nothing else to do, you eat. It becomes your activity of choice. For example, you have nothing to do on Saturday afternoon so you decide to go to the local coffee shop for a latte and scone. You are not hungry. You are bored, seeking some activity. I know some people who take themselves to the movies just so they can enjoy the popcorn. One even told me, "Popcorn is my only joy right now." If you find yourself using food as entertainment, ask yourself what else could be fun? Make a list of activities and places that would be appealing to you. Then set a goal of engaging in one of those activities or going to one of those places this week. Life is about so much more than food but sometimes we lose sight of that.

***Today:* Do a mini-meditation before one meal or snack, eat one meal or snack mindfully and meditate for ten minutes.**

***Today's Journal Question:* What activities can you participate in to replace using food as entertainment?**

FEBRUARY 28:

GOLDEN ARCHES—YOU WANT FRIES WITH THAT?

Back in the 1990s, I had the great fortune to go to Kenya on a photographic safari. It was a bucket list adventure and one that I recommend to everyone to take if they have the chance. My trip began in Nairobi, the capital of Kenya. My travel companions and I spent a day there before traveling to the bush to photograph the animals. When I was in Nairobi, I was struck by how slim the people were. I don't recall seeing many who were overweight or obese. I also don't recall seeing many fast-food restaurants, food chains or supermarkets. Unlike a typical American or Western European capital city, every corner did not sport a hamburger joint, coffee seller or pizza place. In other words, the Nairobi people were not surrounded by environmental food cues. Environmental cues play a big role in what, when and how much we eat.

Close your eyes for a moment and think about your drive to work. Count the number of places you pass that sell food. Include fast food chains, donut shops, coffee stands, supermarkets, gas stations, and liquor stores. Now think about the billboards you see. How many of them offer tempting treats? We are surrounded by food cues all the time. And don't get me started on TV commercials or magazines ads. Cues priming us to eat are everywhere. If you are not mindful, you can easily eat your way through the day, every day. Today notice the food cues in your environment. They include vending machines, candy dishes on your colleague's desks, donut boxes in the break room and posters on the sides of buses. What happens when you see these cues? Do you want to eat? Do you salivate? Does your tummy grumble? Do thoughts such as "those look good" or "one won't hurt" enter your mind? As you answer these questions, be mindful of how these environmental cues might affect your eating and your weight?

Today: **Do a mini-meditation before one meal or snack, eat one meal or snack mindfully and meditate for ten minutes.**

Today's Journal Question: **In what ways does the environment affect your food choices and eating habits?**

FEBRUARY 29:

SHAMPOO, RISE AND REPEAT

Today is a bonus day we get to enjoy every four years. If today happens to be your birthday, Happy Birthday, and be sure to mindfully celebrate four times more than the rest of us do when we have a birthday! Mindfully enjoy your favorite birthday cake and take a moment to be grateful for the life you have and the years you have been on planet Earth. If it is not your birthday, then mindfully eat whatever you want, take a moment to be grateful for your food and then choose your favorite entry from above and reread it. Observe if this second time around is any different than the first. If it is, how is it different?

***Today:* Do a mini-meditation before one meal or snack, eat one meal or snack mindfully and meditate for ten minutes.**

***Today's Journal Question:* Which entry did you choose to repeat and why?**

March

MARCH 1:

WHAT WILL HAPPEN IF YOU GIVE UP EMOTIONAL EATING?

Eating to cope with difficult or unwanted emotions is a national pastime. We all do it in one way or another. Part of being mindful, with respect to your eating, is becoming mindful of your emotions and how you deal with them. It's okay to eat in response to your emotions occasionally, but it is what you do most of the time that defines your lifestyle and impacts your weight.

When I teach mindful eating and its relationship to emotions, I ask my students, *what would happen if they gave up overeating*? Usually, the response I get is a hushed silence sprinkled with nervous giggles. I pause. I give the group time to settle into their reactions.

Slowly, one brave student raises her hand and says, "If I stop eating when I feel my emotions, I will become overwhelmed by them." Heads nod.

Then another courageous soul offers, "I wouldn't know what else to do." More nods.

Now the group is on a roll and I hear, "Eating is fast and easy. Everything else is too hard." "I don't know how to cope without eating." Or, my favorite: "Emotional eating is the only time I get to eat what want. Why would I want to give that up?" Good question. Maybe you are asking it, too.

When we view emotional eating through the lens of mindfulness, we observe it with curiosity and acceptance. We see it as part of what we do and we come to understand its role in our life as well as its sway over us. There is no judgment, no punishment. No self-recrimination or criticism. It is what it is and you have a choice as to whether to participate or not moment by moment. Emotion by emotion. You don't have to give up emotional eating to be a mindful eater but what I have discovered is that as you become a mindful eater, you do less emotional eating. I wonder if that will be true for you too? To help you along we will increase your daily meditation practice to twelve minutes beginning today because research shows that meditation can reduce emotional eating.

***Today:* Do a mini-meditation before two meals or snacks, eat two meals or snacks mindfully and meditate for twelve minutes.**

***Today's Journal Question:* What would happen if you gave up emotional eating?**

MARCH 2:

WHAT RELATIONSHIP DO YOU WANT TO HAVE WITH FOOD?

Our relationship with food can be as complicated as a relationship with a person. I have heard people describe their relationship with food as "love/hate," "I want more than I am getting," "Why can't I have what I want?" "Why is this hard?" and "I keep trying to break up, but we always get back together again." What is your relationship with food like? How would you describe it? Is it supportive and loving, conflicted and hurtful? More important, what relationship with food would you like to have? Would you like a relationship with food that is defined as loving and kind? Nurturing and supportive? Peaceful and serene? If yes, mindful eating can get you there. One of the promises of mindful eating, and one which I am experiencing myself, is peace with food. The battle ends. No more push/pull, love/hate, or want/deny. With mindful eating your mind and body are in sync. You eat what you want when you want it without judgment or regret. If that sounds good to you, keep practicing mindful eating and you'll find out for yourself what I mean.

***Today:* Do a mini-meditation before two meals or snacks, eat two meals or snacks mindfully and meditate for twelve minutes.**

***Today's Journal Question:* What is your relationship to food like?**

MARCH 3:

STRESS RELIEF THE MINDFUL WAY

I've got good news and I've got bad news. The bad news is stress happens. The good news is you don't have to stress eat to feel better. We all seek relief from our stress. We exercise. We drink. We isolate. We yell. We eat. Eating is one way we soothe our frazzled nerves and offer ourselves relief, it's true. You can continue to eat in response to stress if you want too and sometimes you will. But I have another solution that can help reduce how much stress you feel. It's mindful meditation. That's right. It's the meditation I have been encouraging you to practice all along. Research into mindfulness meditation has proven that a consistent, regular practice reduces stress, tension and anxiety.

There is an entire mindfulness-based course called Mindfulness-Based Stress Reduction (MBSR) created by Dr. Jon Kabat-Zinn that has received critical acclaim. You can find MBSR classes throughout the world and online. Take an MBSR class if you'd like that experience. You can also strengthen your commitment to your current practice and derive the benefits right at home. The more you practice, the better able you will be to handle the stressors in your life. The better able you are to handle your stressors, the less likely you are to eat over them. The less likely you are to eat over them the less likely you are to carry extra weight. It's a win-win-win solution.

***Today:* Do a mini-meditation before two meals or snacks, eat two meals or snacks mindfully and meditate for twelve minutes.**

***Today's Journal Question:* How can you change how you handle your stress?**

MARCH 4:
THIS TOO SHALL PASS

Inherent in mindfulness-based wisdom and Buddhist psychology is the notion of impermanence, the idea that everything is temporary. This means that good things don't last forever and neither do the bad ones. The phrase "this too shall pass" can be very helpful in times of strife and hard times. It can also be useful for mindful eating. Even those of us who have embraced mindful eating for a while and who attempt to be mindful at every opportunity, slip up. Mindless eating during a meeting or excess eating at dinner and ice cream binges before bed happen to the best of us. Perhaps it has happened to you. The good news is that a "slip" such as these does not have to morph into a full-blown setback in your mindful eating practice if you adopt the philosophy of impermanence. Just because you ate excessively today, yesterday or even the day before doesn't mean your eating will go on indefinitely. This too shall pass.

Recognizing that eating episodes like those can end, are only temporary, can offer you relief and a *way back to mindful eating.* When you find yourself sliding down a slippery food-soaked slope, pause, take a breath and direct your attention to your food. Take a moment and admire the food mindfully. See it, smell it, touch it and taste it. Ask yourself if it tastes good.

Ask yourself if you are hungry for it. Ask yourself if you need it to soothe yourself. Then continue eating if you choose. Notice if anything has changed. Perhaps you are eating more slowly. Perhaps you are not eating it all. Perhaps nothing has changed at all. Well, that can't be true because for this moment, you were mindful.

Today: **Do a mini-meditation before two meals or snacks, eat two meals or snacks mindfully and meditate for twelve minutes.**

Today's Journal Question: **What challenges with mindful eating are you experiencing?**

MARCH 5:
RISE AND FALL

Are you breathing? Well, of course you are, duh! What I meant to ask is, are you aware of your breathing? Right now, in this moment? Can you feel the rising and falling of your abdomen or are you breathing from your chest? Stop for a second and follow your breath. Right now. Do it. Rise and fall. Rise and fall. Rise and fall. Watch your belly fill up with air and then release it. Slowly, serenely. Rise and fall. Rise and fall. Do this type of abdominal breathing several times a day, especially when you are feeling stressed out or tired, and enjoy the peacefulness that settles within you. Notice if your eating changes as a result of this practice. If you are a stress eater you will most probably eat less.

Today: **Do a mini-meditation before two meals or snacks, eat two meals or snacks mindfully and meditate for twelve minutes.**

Today's Journal Question: **How does paying attention to your breathing help with your eating habits?**

MARCH 6:
I ONLY KNOW ME FROM THE NECK UP

Food is how we nourish ourselves. How we know to nourish ourselves comes from knowing our body. How we know our body comes from being aware of and being comfortable with it. People who struggle with their weight are often disconnected from their bodies. They don't want to pay attention because they don't like what they might see or feel. They only know themselves from the neck up. Is that you? Is it hard for you to see yourself in a mirror? Do you prefer to undress in the dark? Are you unwilling or unable to accept your body as it is right now? Body acceptance is a key component of mindful eating. You may be wondering what body acceptance has to do with eating. A lot, actually. With mindful eating we are trying to gently learn how to listen to our bodies for guidance. To be able to listen to our body we need to accept, appreciate, and value it and its wisdom. Acceptance of your body in a non-judgmental way will take you far on this journey. To help you become more comfortable with your body and learn to appreciate it, I want to introduce you to the Body Scan Meditation.

In this meditation you lie down, close your eyes and relax. Then you bring your attention to one body part at a time starting with your left foot and working your way up and down both sides of the body, ending with the torso, shoulders and head. As you pause at each body part, spend a moment noticing any sensations, thoughts or feelings that come up. Just notice. Do not judge. After you have reached your head, pause again and feel your entire body. Thank it for anything it shared with you during the Body Scan and for its service to you and your life. When you are ready open your eyes and go on with your day. Try to do the Body Scan once a day. I like to do the Body Scan in bed before I sleep. That might be a nice time for you too.

Today: **Do a mini-meditation before two meals or snacks, eat two meals or snacks mindfully and meditate for twelve minutes.**

Today's Journal Question: **How does doing the Body Scan meditation affect how you feel about your body?**

MARCH 7:
EVEN SKINNY PEOPLE OVEREAT

It may surprise you to know that naturally thin people sometime eat ice cream when they are stressed or chocolate when they are sad. It is not a crime to eat junk food. I know. I used to be lawyer! Emotional eating is part of the human condition, so if you do overeat, please don't beat yourself up. Observe it. Pay attention to it and move on. Like in meditation, when your mind wanders, you gently bring your attention back to your breath. Same with eating. If you overeat, emotionally eat, or mindlessly eat, no worries; just gently bring yourself back to mindfulness. Our goal is to be balanced. That naturally thin person who ate ice cream earlier in the day because she had a fight with her boyfriend, "naturally" ate less dinner because she was most likely less hungry than she would have been had she not eaten the ice cream. That's balanced eating. You can become a balanced eater too. All it takes is awareness and guidance from your Inner Wisdom.

***Today:* Do a mini-meditation before two meals or snacks, eat two meals or snacks mindfully and meditate for twelve minutes.**

***Today's Journal Question:* If you have a naturally thin person in your life, what do you notice about their relationship with food?**

MARCH 8:

MINI-MEDITATION CHECK-IN

About a month ago I introduced you to the mini-meditation. This meditation was offered to help you build your mindful eating skills by taking a quick moment to release tension and become aware of your food before a meal or snack. So, how did you do? Did you remember to do it? If you forgot, you could leave a note by your place setting, in your lunch bag or on your fridge as reminder going forward. If you remembered, how did you do? What did you learn? How did it affect your eating? When I started doing mini-meditations I noticed that I ate my meal or snack slower. That was a huge win for me because I am/was a fast eater. I learned to be a fast eater from my mom. Thanks, Mom! Beginning today, please do mini-meditations three (or more times) a day. The more you practice, the more the benefits. If you haven't been practicing, start with once a day and try to move to two soon. You'll reap the rewards more quickly that way.

***Today:* Do a mini-meditation before three meals or snacks, eat two meals or snacks mindfully and meditate for twelve minutes.**

***Today's Journal Question:* How are mini-meditations changing how you eat your meals or snacks?**

MARCH 9:
THE 100-CALORIE CHALLENGE

I am not one to count calories but there is value in knowing the caloric differences among foods so that you can make an informed choice. Mindful eating is not about counting calories or fat grams or anything else. But it is knowing the approximate nutritional value of one food compared to another. Using calories as a way to compare one food with another was used in the MB-EAT research upon which my TAME Your Appetite programs are based. For the research, participants were asked to do a "500-Calorie Challenge" so that they could see how easy it is to remove excess calories without feeling deprived.

As an exercise for today, consider some of your favorite foods to see if you could eat just a little less and still feel full and satisfied. For example, could you eat one less cookie, order a small latte instead of a large or leave a French fry or two on your plate? And if you did, how would you feel? You don't have to cut anything out, just observe. You did a version of this earlier in your journey. Today we are approaching it with more vigor. Over the next week or so investigate calories. Go to the market and compare brands, package sizes and portion servings. Take special note if you could choose one item over another to cut a few calories without feeling denied of your favorite foods or flavors. In the days and weeks to come we will use what you discover to build your Outer Guidance.

***Today:* Do a mini-meditation before three meals or snacks, eat two meals or snacks mindfully and meditate for twelve minutes.**

***Today's Journal Question:* How can you reduce your food intake without feeling deprived?**

MARCH 10:
DO YOU WANT THAT SUPER-SIZED?

Yesterday you began your investigation into ways to eat fewer calories without feeling deprived. Today we will expand that exploration to portion sizes. When I was a kid, a special treat was going to McDonald's for supper. My folks would order me a hamburger, fries and a coke. It was a rare and delicious indulgence. Today, many of us eat McDonald's (or the like) on a regular basis. That by itself is a questionable habit, but more to the point of today's topic of portion sizes, to get the same-sized burger, fries, and coke that I had as a kid, I would need to order a child's Happy Meal. Today an order of burger and fries is much larger than when McDonald's first came on the scene. Everything is larger. If you go to a secondhand store and find a set of dishes from the 1950s, the dinner plate would be the size of today's salad plate and today's dinner plate would have been a platter back then. The problem with the bigger portion sizes and bigger plates is that they are not congruent with our body's needs. Consequently, we are inadvertently, or mindlessly, eating and drinking more than we require. It's time to adjust.

In order for me to eat the right amount of food, I frequently ask for a child's size order. I do that at Starbucks when I want a hot cocoa. I do that at the movies, when I want popcorn. While most restaurants won't let an adult order off of the kid's menu, many will serve half-portions or appetizer-sized servings of adult entrees. If not, they may cut the full serving in half in the kitchen and present one half to you at the table and place the other half in a take-home container. Sometimes your hunger is big and a full serving is just right. Other times it may be too much. Today, try to figure out how you can get served the right amount. Be creative. Your body will thank you.

Today: **Do a mini-meditation before three meals or snacks, eat two meals or snacks mindfully and meditate for twelve minutes.**

Today's Journal Question: **What can you do to mindfully serve yourself the right size helping of a food?**

MARCH 11:

WHAT WOULD HAPPEN IF YOU GAVE UP OVEREATING?

When mindful eating becomes your new normal, you will seldom overeat. You will get accustomed to matching portion sizes to your hunger. When I tell new Mindful Eating students about this, they are excited. This is what they say they want. But after they think about it a little bit, they cringe. Many of them have spent a lifetime overeating and become nervous at the notion that they will no longer be eating as they used to. Hands pop up and questions surface. "What will I do with myself if I am not eating?" "I will have too much time on my hands, what else will I do?" "Where would my joy come from?" Feelings materialize. Deprivation. Fear. Sadness. These questions and feelings are natural. It's understandable if you have concerns.

Mindful Eating may be a big departure from how you used to eat.

There is another side to the "What Would Happen if You Gave Up Overeating" question. The good side. If you gave up overeating you might lose weight, get healthier, have more energy, feel better about yourself, try new things, have time for new hobbies, go back to school, or meet someone special. Take some time today to think about the pros and cons of your overeating. Next consider the pros and cons of ending overeating. Finally, compare your lists and decide what you want for yourself.

***Today:* Do a mini-meditation before three meals or snacks, eat two meals or snacks mindfully and meditate for twelve minutes.**

***Today's Journal Question:* What would happen if you gave up overeating?**

MARCH 12:
WALK THIS WAY

Are you a couch potato? Or a desk jockey? Is most of your day spent not moving? When I was in private practice, mine sure was. I spent hours every day sitting in my big green chair listening to my clients. I had to make a deliberate effort to move around when I wasn't working. My favorite form of movement is walking. It's easy and doesn't take much effort. How much walking are you doing? When I teach my TAME Your Appetite program, mindful walking is part of the curriculum. With mindful walking, your focus is on each step. You take each step slowly noticing as your foot lifts from the ground and strikes down.

If you join me for TAME, I'll teach you how to do it, but for today all I want you to do is take a walk. Walking is a wonderful stress reducer and mood enhancer. A twenty to thirty-minute walk can make you feel good. When you walk, just walk. No headsets or iPods. Use the time to be with yourself. Let your mind wander and notice where it goes. If you can walk in nature, all the better. If possible, make walking a regular part of your daily life. Your body, mind and spirit will benefit.

***Today:* Do a mini-meditation before three meals or snacks, eat two meals or snacks mindfully and meditate for twelve minutes.**

***Today's Journal Question:* How can you make walking a part of your daily routine?**

MARCH 13:
MINDFUL TASTE EXPERIENCE

Taste is an essential component of Mindful Eating and plays two important roles. First, we want to eat foods that taste good to us. When you begin eating more mindfully and pay closer attention to how foods taste, you may discover that some foods you eat frequently don't really taste that good. That can happen if you have been a quick eater or a mindless one. You just chew and swallow without actually tasting the food. With mindful eating, you pay attention to the taste of food and if a food does not taste good you may choose not to consume it. Because of mindful eating you have the "presence of mind" to notice and make such a choice. The second role taste plays has to do with deciding to stop eating. Taste changes as we eat. The first few bites of something are the most flavorful. A few bites later our taste buds are less sensitive to the taste and the taste decreases. This decrease in taste can be used as factor in considering when to stop eating.

You can choose to stop as soon as a food's taste diminished or choose to enjoy a few more bites and then end. I notice a taste change most readily with chewing gum. I often enjoy a small piece of mint gum after a meal or snack. Within minutes the gum has lost most of its favor and I toss it out. With mindful eating you no longer stop eating simply because there is no more food on the plate. When to stop eating is a decision you will now make mindfully. When you eat today, pay special attention to taste. Do you like how a particular food tastes? What might make it taste better? A bit of salt? Toasting it? Cooling it off? If a food does not taste good to you, ask yourself if you want to keep eating it. Observe how you make your decision. Also, notice when the taste changes.

Today: **Do a mini-meditation before three meals or snacks, eat two meals or snacks mindfully and meditate for twelve minutes.**

Today's Journal Question: **What role does taste play in your eating habits?**

MARCH 14:
I CAN'T GET NO SATISFACTION

Have you ever had the experience when no matter how much you ate you weren't satisfied? You'd order more at a restaurant or finished all the food on your plate even though you weren't hungry anymore? Or if you are at home, you'd keep opening the refrigerator door peering in to see if anything appealed to you. Or maybe you're out and find yourself walking the aisles of a supermarket looking for whatever might "do the trick"? If you find yourself wanting to eat when you are not hungry, you are sliding into mindless or emotional eating. When you notice you are eating past the point of satisfaction or fullness, ask yourself why this might be happening. (Or if you become aware of this later, ask yourself the same question.) Think back and review the thoughts, feelings and behaviors leading up to the excess eating. Were you socializing? Did an emotion arise such as fear or sadness? Were you bored? Was the food just there? A bit of mindful detective work can uncover the reason for the eating. When you uncover your why, note it. Reflect upon it non-judgmentally. Be curious about the chain of events that got you there. What can you learn from this insight? How can you use this insight in the future? File this incident away and move on. Demonstrate love and kindness to yourself by eating your next meal mindfully.

***Today:* Do a mini-meditation before three meals or snacks, eat two meals or snacks mindfully and meditate for twelve minutes.**

***Today's Journal Question:* How do you know when you are satisfied by what you ate?**

MARCH 15:
WOULD YOU LIKE CREAM OR SUGAR WITH THAT?

About two months ago, you did an exercise where you tried a new food. The purpose of that exercise was to get you into the habit of trying new things and really tasting them. Now I would like you to do the same with beverages. Like with your food choices, you may be stuck in a drink-rut, choosing the same latte at the coffee shop or cold drink at the deli. Such habitual choices are another form of mindless consumption. Becoming a mindful eater means being a mindful drinker too. For today I would like you to go to the market or coffee shop or deli (wherever) and buy a new drink. Like when you did this exercise with food, find a location where you can drink it without interruption. And like before, try to be a little bit hungry.

When you are settled in the location where you will drink your drink, take a moment to get centered. Adjust your seating so you are comfortable. Turn off all electronics. Take a few deep breaths. And, when you are ready, turn your attention to your beverage and do the following:

- Look at it. Notice its color.

- Bring it to your nose and take a long deep inhale. Notice its scent.
- Bring it to your lips and take a single sip.
- Imagine you are tasting the finest beverage ever made.
- Notice its flavor.
- Savor the flavor.
- When you are ready, swallow.
- Drink your beverage one sip at a time savoring each.
- Really notice the flavor.
- Stop when you've had enough, or it stops tasting good, or it's gone.

When you are finished ask yourself if this is a beverage you might like to add to your repertoire of choices. If yes, why yes? If no, why not? Try to do this exercise once a month to help you explore new beverages and build your mindful eating skills. You never know you might just discover a new favorite!

***Today:* Do a mini-meditation before three meals or snacks, eat two meals or snacks mindfully and meditate for twelve minutes.**

***Today's Journal Question:* Describe your experience of mindfully enjoying a new beverage.**

MARCH 16:
ALL FOODS ARE "LEGAL"

You may not know this about me but my first career was as an attorney. If you have been to law school you know it can be challenging. If you ever watched the movie The Paper Chase you would know what my first day of law school was like. Just like Timothy Button's character, James Hart, I, too, was the first person asked a question using the Socratic Method by my Torts professor on the first day of class (for Hart it was contract law.) And like Hart, I felt unprepared and stupid. Tough way to start off. I learned a lot in law school. But one thing I didn't learn was that all foods are "legal." No, when I was in law school, I dieted. All kinds of diets. Those were the days before I understood that diets are not the way to go to manage my weight (or my emotions). It wasn't until I truly embraced mindful eating that I accepted this truth and my relationship with food changed for the better. What do I mean when I say that all foods are legal? I mean that you are welcome to choose from all the foods available in the world to meet your physical hunger. When you are mindful this is quite easy to do.

You are not limited to a food list or specific combinations. You decide based on your body's needs. This idea may seem scary, especially if you have relied on diet plans for a long time. But try it. Today, when you are hungry, ask yourself what you would prefer to eat. Choose exactly what you want and then prepare, serve and eat it mindfully. Savor the colors, smells and taste. Notice when you feel full and how eating that particular food felt for your body. As you practice eating "legal" foods, you may find yourself gravitating towards food you previously avoided. That's okay. Enjoy yourself. Mindfully, of course. If you are like me, and others I have worked with, after a while "legalized foods" become ordinary. They fall in line with other foods that were always permissible. They lose their "charge" and in time you can take them or leave them. Now that's what I call peace with food!

***Today:* Do a mini-meditation before three meals or snacks, eat two meals or snacks mindfully and meditate for twelve minutes.**

***Today's Journal Question:* What thoughts and feeling show up when you think about making all food legal?**

MARCH 17:
HOW MANY LIKES DO YOU HAVE?

Thanks to Facebook we now go around thinking in terms of likes and dislikes. We are quick to give something or someone a thumbs-up or down based on our opinion. The same is true for our opinion of food. Some foods we give a thumbs-up. Others thumbs-down. How do you decide which food gets which response? Before mindful eating, you may have based your opinion of food on whether it was "on your diet" or "if it will make you fat" or "if it will make you thin." With mindful eating, your approach is different. You now make such a choice without these judgments. Food is food. None of it is all bad and none of it is all good. It depends. It depends on you.

To arrive at the place where food is food, you start by acknowledging your response to food without judgment. In other words, if you think that hot fudge sundaes are the devil's work, notice that. Do not judge yourself for having this opinion. It's just an opinion. Approach it now as you do with most things, with curiosity and acceptance. You are not bad for having this opinion, nor are you good. When you can experience your beliefs about food without judgment and when you become neutral about your food choices, you will no longer be obligated to rules. You will be free to make mindful decisions based on what is right for you at that moment. And, sometimes, a hot fudge sundae is exactly right.

Today: Do a mini-meditation before three meals or snacks, eat two meals or snacks mindfully and meditate for twelve minutes.

Today's Journal Question: What happens when you approach food without judgment?

MARCH 18:

NO MORE SHOULDS

Shoulda, woulda, coulda. The constant refrain of how we ought to be feeling, thinking, and acting. Feel this way, don't feel that way. Think this thought, not that one. Eat this, don't eat that! When you adopt mindfulness as the fabric of your life, this refrain changes to feel as you feel, think as you think, and eat as you eat. The ultimate "should" when it comes to eating is the United States Department of Agriculture's Food Pyramid (called MyPyramid) which was created to provide nutritional recommendations of the kinds and amounts of food to each day. While a good idea in theory, the problem is we are all different and recommendations for one person may be not be right for another. With the mindful eating skills you are learning, you don't need the USDA Food Pyramid (or the more recent version, MyPlate) to tell you what to eat. Your body will guide you to what is right for you. Feel free to use MyPyramid and MyPlate as information to inform your choices, but let your body take the lead.

***Today:* Do a mini-meditation before three meals or snacks, eat two meals or snacks mindfully and meditate for twelve minutes**

***Today's Journal Question:* How can you let your body take the lead in what you eat instead of relying on the USDA MyPlate?**

MARCH 19:

TAKE YOURSELF OUT TO DINNER

When someone in my clinical psychology practice was struggling with a breakup and they were having a hard time getting on with their life, I would recommend that they take themselves on a date. I suggested they treat themselves the way they would want to be treated on a date—flowers, fancy dinner, the works. Later, as I broadened my work to include mindful eating, I made a similar recommendation to my mindful eating clients, take yourself out to dinner. The recommendation was the same, but the reason was different. For the heartbroken, it was to rebuild their self-esteem.

For the mindful eater, it was to have the experience of really dining, not just eating. We all go out to eat. Some of us multiple times a day or week. But do you dine when you eat out? Do you get served? Do you linger over the menu? Do you savor the dessert? Or do you just eat? This week, I want you to take yourself (and a loved one if you like) out to dinner. It doesn't have to be fancy or expensive but choose a place where you order and dine at a table. If the table has a cloth on it—even better. Try to get to the restaurant a bit hungry, but not too hungry. Just hungry enough to be ready for a meal.

Then, when you are seated, take a moment to look at the décor. Take in the ambiance of the place. Notice the colors, sights and sounds. Observe the other diners. Next, before you open the menu, check in with yourself. Ask yourself what you would like to eat. Hot or cold? Light or hearty? Crunchy or creamy? Then open the menu. Pursue each item on the menu. Imagine how they might taste. Listen intently if the server explains specials of the day. When you are ready, place your order choosing what you really want to eat and not what you think you should. If there is bread on the table and you want some, have some. Eat it mindfully, savoring each morsel.

When your meal comes, thank the server and silently thank all the others who participated in bringing this meal to you. Now, enjoy your meal. Eat the first bite like you did the raisin long ago. Delight in the food in front of you. Check in with your fullness as you go along. If you are full before the food is gone, set it aside. Ask for a take-home container if you wish. If you want dessert, save room for it. When the meal is over, acknowledge yourself for a wonderful evening. Pat yourself on the back for your mindfulness. When you get home, journal about the experience and how it was different than how you usually eat out.

***Today:* Do a mini-meditation before three meals or snacks, eat two meals or snacks mindfully and meditate for twelve minutes.**

***Today's Journal Question:* Enjoy a restaurant meal and describe your experience.**

MARCH 20:
THE INTERCONNECTEDNESS OF ALL LIFE

There is an app you might like called Insight Timer. You can get it for free on your iPhone. On it are thousands of meditations of all types, lengths and teachers. There are two features that I especially love about this app. The first is that it tells you how many people are meditating around the world at the same time you are. For example, I just logged on and at this moment there are 2,464 people meditating using the app and so far, 219,855 people have meditated today. How awesome is that? The second feature I love is that you can connect with friends through it. One of my MB-EAT colleagues lives in Australia. Because we are friends on Insight Timer, I can see when she is meditating, and we can plan to meditate together—all the way across the world!

An unexpected and tremendous gift I got from adopting mindfulness and mindful eating is the sense of being connected to everything and everyone on the planet. This happened because one element of mindful eating is being aware of and expressing gratitude to all who contributed to the food we eat. For instance, recognizing all the people who participated in bringing me the orange I ate for my morning snack, as well as all the elements of nature required to grow it, makes me feel connected to the world around me. We are not alone when we are mindful. We are all interconnected. If you eat because you are lonely, use mindfulness to remind yourself that you, too, are interconnected to all there is. That you and I are linked to each other even though we have yet to meet.

Today: **Do a mini-meditation before three meals or snacks, eat two meals or snacks mindfully and meditate for twelve minutes.**

Today's Journal Question: **With whom are you connected?**

MARCH 21:
BEING AT EASE WITH FOOD

A great joy that comes from mindful eating is the ability to be at ease with food. What do I mean by that? I mean that because of mindful eating you will be comfortable in the presence of food. Regardless of where you are, what is being served or not being served, you will be just fine. When you are dieting, the world is a harder place to navigate. How many times have you turned down an invitation because you were afraid of the food? Afraid that there won't be anything you can eat on your diet. Afraid that you will be tempted by what is being offered that you will overeat. How many times have you ordered a plain green salad, dressing on the side, while others in your party were enjoying a nice steak or pasta dish? How many times did you say "the heck with it" and throw caution to the wind and overindulge because you were tired of being on a diet? If you are a chronic dieter, I'm guessing your answer will be "a lot."

Now, imagine having the confidence that wherever you go you know in your heart that you will make the right decisions about food. Imagine that you can enjoy a steak or pasta dish, eating exactly the correct amount for you and taking the rest home for later. Imagine having dressing on your salad if that is how you like it or choosing a salad instead of pizza because you want a salad. By tuning into your internal cues (like hunger, taste and fullness) you can do just that. When you take your mindful eating habits with you, you can go anywhere. Food becomes easy. It becomes a non-issue. How cool is that?

***Today:* Do a mini-meditation before three meals or snacks, eat two meals or snacks mindfully and meditate for twelve minutes.**

***Today's Journal Question:* What does being at ease with food mean to you?**

MARCH 22:
THE MINDFUL RECIPE

Playing on the TV at my local nail salon is the Food Channel. It doesn't matter what time of day or day of the week I have my appointment; the Food Channel is on. Over the years I have seen snippets of the shows that air on that channel but I was never one to really watch, until I became mindful. While my nails were being filed and my toes were soaking in the pedicure tub, I focused my attention on the TV screen and saw that a pasta entrée was being prepared. This time instead of poking my head up from my book to catch a glimpse, I closed my book and paid full attention. I watched as the chef carefully measured out each ingredient for the dish. I observed her hands as she skillfully cut the vegetables into bite-sized pieces and tossed them into boiling water. I listened as she described the best way to cook pasta and how to toss it so all the noodles are evenly coated with sauce. I studied her beautiful table setting complete with ceramic dishware and colorful napkins. I could almost smell the aroma of the dish as she placed it on the table.

When I returned home from the nail salon, I was motivated to make pasta for dinner and to do as she did. I carefully prepared my ingredients, took great pleasure in chopping, dicing and slicing. I admired the colors and flavors as they revealed themselves and inhaled deeply as the scent of the tomato sauce wafting through my kitchen. I set a beautiful table, using some special china I rarely take out and mindfully ate my dinner. Have you ever made a dish from scratch? Have you done so with your full attention? Try it. Mindfully engage in each step of the process. Don't distract yourself with music or television. Just be there with your recipe and its ingredients. And when you are done, mindfully enjoy your creation with all your senses.

Today: **Do a mini-meditation before three meals or snacks, eat two meals or snacks mindfully and meditate for twelve minutes.**

Today's Journal Question: **Describe your experience of mindfully preparing a recipe.**

MARCH 23:

MINDFUL WATER AEROBICS

In YMCAs across the country, people gather in the shallow end of the swimming pool for water aerobics. These classes are not as athletic as they sound but they sure are fun! Once week, I attend such a class at my local gym. I love being in the water, splashing, kicking, and running in place. One morning while I was waiting for the class to begin, I wondered what it would be like if I made the water my focus. Could I do a water aerobics meditation?

I was at a point in my meditation practice where I was experimenting with different focal points for my attention besides my breath. Sometimes I used sound. Other times I used the flicker of a candle. Today I wondered if I could use the water. I have been to this class so many times that I pretty much knew the routine, so I was confident I could divert my attention from the teacher to the water. And I did. As the class got started, I felt the water against my skin, a bit chilly but oh so smooth.

Then, as we moved in rhythm to the music, I watched the water ripple and bubble. I saw waves crest and crash like a tempest storm as our movements got more intense and then settle down as still as a lake when we stopped to stretch. Whenever my mind wandered from the water (and it did, of course) I gently brought myself back to the water. You want to know where my thoughts wandered to? To you my dear reader, to you. I kept thinking about how I would explain to you what I was experiencing. Each time my thoughts drifted to you, I noted it, labeling the thought as "reader" and then reminded myself to return to the water. By the time the class finished I was convinced this was the best form of meditation out there! The next time you are in a pool, or doing any form of exercise for that matter, find something to place your attention on and practice the skill of returning to your reference point when your mind wanders. You can thank me later!

***Today:* Do a mini-meditation before three meals or snacks, eat two meals or snacks mindfully and meditate for twelve minutes.**

***Today's Journal Question:* When can you practice the skill of returning your mind to a point of reference?**

MARCH 24:

BEGIN AGAIN . . . AND AGAIN . . . AND AGAIN . . .

Meditation is all about beginning again. When your mind wanders you begin again by bringing your attention back to the breath. You do this as many times as you need too. Back to the breath. Back to the beginning. This is the practice. Mindful eating is also about beginning again and again as many times as you need. Whenever you eat mindlessly or eat from your emotions you have the opportunity to begin again. Simply redirect your focus to mindful eating with the next plateful, forkful, lick or bite. Simply begin again. There is no judgement. No criticism. Only observation. Awareness and the decision to begin again. How fortunate are we that we can always begin again?

***Today:* Do a mini-meditation before three meals or snacks, eat two meals or snacks mindfully and meditate for twelve minutes.**

***Today's Journal Question:* When in your life did you begin again?**

MARCH 25:

MINDFUL GROCERY SHOPPING

Do you charge through the grocery store, tossing items into your cart and then hustle your way back to the car happy to be done with this chore?

Or when you shop, do you have kids in tow, clamoring for one food product after another resulting in an unwelcomed power struggle that usually ends with someone in tears? Or do you enjoy grocery shopping? Do you take your time and leisurely walk up and down the aisles admiring the great selection of food stuffs we have to choose from? If you haven't, that is your assignment for today (or Sunday, whenever).

Take yourself on a mindful grocery shopping trip. Give yourself an hour or two to visit a market. It could be your usual store or one you rarely frequent. You could pick the 24-hour joint on the corner or an ethnic shop on the other side of town. Choose a destination that is interesting to you. When you arrive, turn your cellphone on silent, put away any lists or coupons, grab a basket and just meander. Use all your senses to experience the ambiance around you. Pick up products you haven't seen before and read their labels. If something appeals to you, put it in your basket. Wander up and down the aisles. Notice your reactions to the foods you see. What are you thinking? Feeling? Do not judge yourself, just observe. Be mindful of your surroundings. When you are finished, pay for the items you placed in your basket knowing that you made mindful choices, and then take a moment to reflect on how this shopping trip is different than your weekly runs. Is there anything you could do more mindfully the next time you are in the store? When you are ready, mindfully drive home.

***Today:* Do a mini-meditation before three meals or snacks, eat two meals or snacks mindfully and meditate for twelve minutes.**

***Today's Journal Question:* Describe your most recent shopping experience in terms of mindfulness and mindlessness.**

MARCH 26:

YOU'RE THE BOSS

Back in the 1980s and 90s there was a hit TV show called *Who's The Boss?* The sitcom starred Judith Light as Angela, a working single mom, and Tony Danza as Tony, her housekeeper. In keeping with its name, the show centered on the humorous power struggle between Angela and Tony as to who was really in charge of the household. You may be having the same struggle (although maybe not as funny) with yourself as to what, when, and how much to eat. You know by now that a guiding principle in mindful eating is the freedom to choose foods based on your own needs. This freedom can feel perilous to those who do not yet trust themselves in this regard. The structure of a diet can seem comforting when you are in the midst of mindless eating but I assure you that in the long run trusting yourself to guide you will serve you better than some random diet.

As you learn to understand your body's signals and which foods work best for you, you will develop this trust I am talking about. As you progress with your mindful eating journey, please keep in mind that there is no right or wrong way to eat, only your way. Know, too, that your dietary needs might fluctuate day to day, life phase to life phase, as will your degrees of awareness regarding your eating habits and food preferences. Your eating experiences will vary and each one will be unique in its one way. Ultimately you will make choices that support your health and well-being and when asked, "Who's the Boss?" the answer will be resoundingly—you.

Today: **Do a mini-meditation before three meals or snacks, eat two meals or snacks mindfully and meditate for twelve minutes.**

Today's Journal Question: **Who (or what) is the boss over you and why?**

MARCH 27:
MINDFUL MUSIC

I enjoy the opera. I don't go very often but when I do go, I love the whole experience. What is most meaningful to me about an opera is the emotional connection I feel with the music. The performers may be singing in a language I don't understand but if I close my eyes and let the music fill me up, I can feel the meaning of their words. You may not be an opera buff but I suspect there are genres of music that you love to listen to. (I also love disco—please don't hold that against me!)

As an exercise in mindfulness, choose a song you especially like and listen to it purposefully. Set aside time to be alone. Put in earbuds. Sit. Take a few deep breathes and listen. Really listen. Close your eyes and hear the lyrics. If there are no lyrics, concentrate on the melody and allow yourself to fully experience it. What do you feel? If there are lyrics, pay attention to the actual words being sung. Do they mean anything to you? Do they resonate with you? Listen to the song again, shifting your attention from the lyrics to the melody. Can you feel it in your body? Are you experiencing any emotions? Memories? Thoughts? Play your song over a few times so you really get into it. If you want to move, dance, or sing along, do that. Attend to the music with intention and purpose and notice if doing so makes this encounter more pleasurable than when you've heard it before. Mindfully listening to a piece of music can be an enriching and satisfying activity.

***Today:* Do a mini-meditation before three meals or snacks, eat two meals or snacks mindfully and meditate for twelve minutes.**

***Today's Journal Question:* After mindfully listening to some music, reflect on your experience.**

MARCH 28:

DO YOU KNOW YOUR SWEET SPOT?

Learning to assess how full you are is an essential component of mindful eating. Up until now you have been working with your awareness of your hunger. Now it is time to figure out when you are full. You probably know when you are uncomfortably full. The "I can't believe I ate the whole thing" feeling. That feeling usually shows up as a result of mindless eating. There is a fullness sweet spot. The spot when you have eaten enough food to meet your body's needs and you don't need to unbuckle your belt. When you eat beyond that sweet spot you are taking in more food than your body needs and that typically leads to excess weight. Tuning into your fullness sweet spot and learning to stop eating when you get there will prevent overeating and get you to the right weight for you. So, how do you find your sweet spot? By now, you probably can guess the answer—by being mindful!

Check in with yourself while you are eating to judge how full you are. It might be helpful to create a Fullness Awareness Scale as a gauge. We use such a scale in some of TAME programs. You could imagine that a one on your Fullness Awareness Scale is "not full at all" and a ten is as full as "a binge might leave you." Your sweet spot is most likely around a five or six. Beginning today, practice with your Fullness Awareness Scale. See how much food you eat to reach your sweet spot. Remember this amount will change based on what your body requires in any given moment. You don't have to stop eating when you reach your sweet spot if you are not ready to build that skill. Just be aware of where your sweet spot is and how you feel if you stop eating and how you feel if you continue eating.

***Today:* Do a mini-meditation before three meals or snacks, eat two meals or snacks mindfully and meditate for twelve minutes.**

Today's Journal Question: **How does your body let you know when you are comfortably full?**

MARCH 29:
THE FULLNESS CONUNDRUM

I hope that you have been practicing the skill of Mindful Fullness and as a result you are getting better at knowing when your body has had enough to eat. Have you also practiced stopping eating when you are full? For many, that part is harder than knowing when you are full. If you are struggling with discontinuing eating when you know you have had enough, you are not alone. The question I have for you is, "Why do you keep eating after fullness?" Among the answers I hear to that question are (1) "it's delicious, I don't want to stop," (2) "I never get to eat this food, so I want to eat it all," and (3) "if I stop now, I'll be hungry later." Are any of these answers your answer? My response to the first two is the same. You can always have this food again—when you are hungry. This is not your very last time. The next time you are hungry, serve it up. Serve it up every time you are hungry. Not a problem. If it is your very last time because, for example, you are in a foreign country you plan to never visit again, then eat it all—mindfully. Relish every last morsel. Lick the plate if you like. Mindful eating is about enjoying your food, so enjoy. This is a special occasion, just remember, not every meal is special.

As for the third answer, I want to introduce you to another component of Mindful Fullness, an advanced skill if you will, the skill of recognizing how long your fullness last and which foods are more filling for you at which times. To learn this skill, pay attention to which foods keep you fuller longer. For example, if you know that you will not have a chance to eat again until five or six hours after your breakfast, you might choose a more filling breakfast. You could eat more of what you usually eat, or you could eat something different. Perhaps a bowl of oatmeal with a swirl of peanut butter in it will hold you better than jam on toast. The more you practice these skills, more you improve and the sooner they will become second nature to you.

Today: **Do a mini-meditation before three meals or snacks, eat two meals or snacks mindfully and meditate for twelve minutes.**

Today's Journal Question: **What thoughts and feelings arise when you think about not eating when you are full?**

MARCH 30:

THE 15-MINUTE BUMP

It's time to bump up your meditation practice to fifteen minutes. If you are ready, use a guided meditation recording from an app or CD. Try different guided meditations to learn what you like. If you don't want to use a guided meditation, you can set a timer for fifteen minutes and go on your own. Do whatever serves you best. Make this practice your own.

If you are not ready, acknowledge yourself for the efforts you have been making so far. If you are still not doing any meditation, reflect on why not. What is getting in your way? Try not to be harsh with yourself. Investigate what is going on from a position of non-judgment and self-compassion. It is hard to do something new. Meditation can seem scary to some people, maybe you.

If you are really struggling, find a meditation class in your area. Many universities and yoga studios offer meditation classes. That's how I started. Some places have drop-in sessions where you can come and go as you please. Others offer meditation series lasting six to eight weeks.

Whatever you are doing, or not doing, is okay. Kindness towards yourself is your best bolster.

If you are practicing continue at least six times during the week keeping track of your meditation practice in your journal.

***Today:* Do a mini-meditation before three meals or snacks, eat two meals or snacks mindfully and meditate for fifteen minutes.**

***Today's Journal Question:* What can you do to support yourself as you increase the length of your daily meditation practice?**

MARCH 31:

REVIEW TIME—HOW FAR HAVE YOU COME?

Welcome to the end of month three of your journey to mindful eating. I hope you have been enjoying it and that your foundational meditation practice is solidifying. It is time now to check in and see which benefits of mindful eating and meditation you are already receiving. Are you:

1. More tuned into your hunger signals?
2. More aware of when you are full?
3. Able to end eating even with food on your plate?

4. More mindful of what and how much to eat?
5. Choosing foods you enjoy and taste good to you?
6. Eating less?
7. Noticing any improvement in your relationship with food?
8. Are you feeling more relaxed around food?
9. Able to bring your attention back to your breath when your mind wanders?
10. Sitting for longer periods during your meditation sessions?
11. Feeling less stressed?
12. Feeling less anxious?
13. Doing less emotional or binge eating?
14. Looking forward to your meditation sessions?
15. Losing weight?

Check in with these questions periodically to see your movement forward.

***Today:* Do a mini-meditation before three meals or snacks, eat two meals or snacks mindfully and meditate for fifteen minutes.**

***Today's Journal Question:* What changes are you noticing since beginning your journey to mindful eating?**

APRIL

◆◆◆

APRIL 1:
THE PRINCIPLES OF MINDFULNESS

Mindful eating is not new. The tradition of mindfulness is thousands of years old. We in the Western world are rediscovering it and adapting it to our modern culture. That being said, it is valuable to take a look at the principles behind mindfulness to see how they inform our work in mindful eating and contemporary mindfulness in general. There are seven principles of mindfulness. They are: non-judging; patience; non-striving; letting go; acceptance; beginner's mind; and trust. Each one plays a role in mindful eating and mindful meditation. In the days to come we will explore each one in depth.

We will look at how trust, patience and non-striving can support you as you give up dieting and embrace the mindful approach. Exploring what a beginner's mind is will show us how to avoid relapsing into binges or giving up completely. Letting go, non-judging and acceptance will play a role in minimizing reactivity which could lead to trashing this approach and signing up for another diet. After these principles, we will also look at three other mindfulness ideas that support mindful eating. Those are self-compassion, impermanence and non-attachment to outcome. You don't need to be a Buddhist or believe in Eastern philosophy to benefits from these ideas. Simply be open-minded and curious as we explore how these principles can benefit you.

Today: **Do a mini-meditation before three meals or snacks, eat two meals or snacks mindfully and meditate for fifteen minutes.**

Today's Journal Question: **How can being open-minded and curious about the Principles of Mindfulness serve you?**

APRIL 2:
TRUST, PATIENCE AND NON-STRIVING

Becoming a mindful eater can, in many ways, be seen as a leap of faith. Having spent years, maybe even decades, relying on diets to gain control over your eating, you may be feeling a drift with the idea of taking this non-diet approach. The Buddhist traditions of trust, patience and non-striving will serve you well here. Let's look at how each can help you on your journey. Trust supports you in two ways. First, you can trust the idea that your body knows what is best for your health and well-being. Your body is a magnificent creation that engages in multiple of processes that keep us alive. How can an entity so sophisticated and miraculous steer you wrong? Second, you can trust the science behind mindfulness-based eating, MB-EAT, upon which my approach to mindful eating is based, because it is an evidence-based protocol with decades of solid research behind it. This is not a fly-by-night approach. You can depend on it.

Next, patience sustains you because this approach takes time. Unlike crash diets where you may see results quickly, mindful eating shows its benefits over time. Stick with it and you too will reap its rewards. Lastly, non-striving encourages you to relax into this process rather than forcing it to happen. You don't have to try so hard to gain results. Unlike diets, food rules or expert opinions which perpetuate your weight and eating problems by adding stress to the mix, mindful eating is the peaceful way to go. Practice these three principles and you will see for yourself how they carry you along this journey.

***Today:* Do a mini-meditation before three meals or snacks, eat two meals or snacks mindfully and meditate for fifteen minutes.**

***Today's Journal Question:* How can trust, patience and non-striving serve you as you develop your mindful eating habits?**

APRIL 3:
YOUR "BEGINNER'S MIND"

You may have heard the phrase "beginner's mind" before now. It is frequently talked about in the world of meditation and in Buddhist teachings. To have a "beginner's mind" means to approach life unencumbered by previous knowledge and experience. Even seasoned meditators practice "beginner's mind." When you come to a meditation or any task with a "beginner's mind" you undertake it as if for the first time. The task is new and fresh. Having a "beginner's mind" will serve you well in your journey to mindful eating because it asks you to release all previous expectations, experiences and ideas. It allows you to respond in a new spontaneous way to what is happening around you. This will be especially useful to avoid turning a slip of mindless eating into a full-blown binge or to prevent a lapse in your meditation practice from becoming a signal to quit. "Beginner's mind" takes away thoughts like, "Here we go again. I never stick to a plan. This doesn't work either." "I already ate ten cookies might as well finish the whole box." And, "My mind keeps wandering, this meditation stuff isn't for me."

These thoughts reflect opinions based on history. With a "beginner's mind" there is no history, there is only now. What happened before doesn't matter. And more important it does not have to happen again. You have choice with "beginner's mind." You have the choice to respond with curiosity rather than condemnation. So, instead of assuming that having a slip is the same as failing or ten cookies equals a whole box or a wandering mind means you can't meditate, observe what is happening with inquisitiveness. Are you sure you never stick to plan? Is it possible to stop at ten cookies? Could a wandering mind be useful? Seeing life with a "beginner's mind" brings back the wonders of childhood. Try it. You may like it.

Today: Do a mini-meditation before three meals or snacks, eat two meals or snacks mindfully and meditate for fifteen minutes.

Today's Journal Question: In what ways can you practice having a "beginner's mind"?

APRIL 4:
LETTING GO, NON-JUDGING AND ACCEPTANCE

Now we will turn to the next three Principles of Mindfulness: Letting go, non-judging and acceptance. Personally, I stress these three principles in the work I do with all my clients. When I can help them to let go of preconceived notions and ideas, to stop judging themselves and to accept themselves and those around them, I go a long way in guiding them to mindfulness. Think about this for a moment. Imagine how calm you might feel if you stop expecting, judging and forcing things to go your way. Try this. Clutch your fists as hard as you can. Really tight. Tighter. Tighter. Feel the tension and strain around your fingers and knuckles. Now open them up. Do you feel a rush of energy as you release your grip? Do your hands feel more relaxed?

That release, that flow of calmness can be yours when you learn to let go, not judge and accept. These three principles will work together to calm weight-related anxieties based on expectations, judgment and force by assisting you in cultivating a point-of-view that avoids reactivity and allows for thoughtful action. By learning to be less reactive you can prevent the urge to toss this approach and go in search of another diet. Instead, you will stay the course and graduate to mindful eating.

T*oday:* Do a mini-meditation before three meals or snacks, eat two meals or snacks mindfully and meditate for fifteen minutes.

***Today's Journal Question:* Of the three principles, which one might prove to be the most difficult for you to cultivate and why?**

APRIL 5:

MIRROR, MIRROR WHO'S THE FAIREST OF THEM ALL?

Grab a hand mirror or walk over to a wall mirror and look at your reflection. Is that easy or hard for you to do? Do you shy away from your reflection? I am here to tell you that the reflection in the mirror deserves your love. It deserves your compassion. Self-compassion is an important mindfulness concept. Whole books and meditation programs have been created about it. In this journey, we will use self-compassion to guide you to be patient with yourself and this process. So often we are impatient, punitive and self-critical. We demand more of ourselves than we do of others.

This harshness is the opposite of self-compassion and can derail our efforts for self-improvement. What we need is a form of loving kindness towards ourselves. When we are kind rather than critical of ourselves, we can do and be more. Today treat yourself as you would a dear friend. Speak to yourself as you would speak to an elderly relative. Nurture yourself as you would a sweet child. You deserve it.

***Today:* Do a mini-meditation before three meals or snacks, eat two meals or snacks mindfully and meditate for fifteen minutes.**

***Today's Journal Question:* What act of kindness can you offer yourself today?**

APRIL 6:

NOTHING LASTS FOREVER

Impermanence is another aspect of mindfulness which will be used as you become a mindful eater. Impermanence teaches us that everything (including our weight) is temporary. Impermanence can be a challenging concept to grasp because no one really wants to think about things ending. But endings are often good and they are inevitable. Nothing lasts forever as much as we might want it to. In a way we can say that everything is temporary. Day is temporary because it turns to night. Spring is temporary because it turns to summer. Relying on this idea, excess weight can be seen as a temporary state. It, too, can transition into something else. You were not always this weight, were you?

You may be carrying extra weight today, but a year from now your weight can be different. We can approach binges and emotional eating episodes the same way. They don't last forever. You do stop eating. You do regain control and get back to mindfulness. Keeping impermanence in mind can help end the "I've blown it, this will never work, might as well eat it all" mentality. Sure, we all may want the good stuff to go on indefinitely but we can take comfort in knowing that the bad stuff ends, too.

***Today:* Do a mini-meditation before three meals or snacks, eat two meals or snacks mindfully and meditate for fifteen minutes.**

***Today's Journal Question:* What in your life is temporary and that's a good thing?**

APRIL 7:
WHATEVER WILL BE WILL BE (QUE SERA SERA)

When I was a kid in the late 1960s, Doris Day had a television show, and its theme song was "Que Sera Sera (Whatever Will Be Will Be)." I loved that song. The lyrics told the story of the singer's life as it progressed from childhood to teens to adulthood. At each stage, the singer asked questions about what her life would be like. The answer was always the same: "What will be, will be." What a perfect lyric to express the mindfulness idea of Non-Attachment to Outcomes. Non-attachment to outcomes means that while we may covet a certain result, we are okay if it doesn't come. Being okay if our desired result doesn't come can reduce the suffering that impatience causes. In this mindful eating journey, it means allowing your process to unfold its own natural way, the way that is best for you and your body. To help you understand this better, think back to a diet you were on.

While dieting, you probably based your success on what the scale said. If you lost weight that week, you were "good"; if you didn't you were "bad." This is very common. As a society, we are so attached to the number on the scale that we lose sight of the many other successes that actually occurred that week. For example, maybe we didn't eat when we weren't hungry, we stopped when we were full, we said no to seconds, we meditated daily, we expressed our emotions instead of eating over them, or we showed up for ourselves in ways we might not have before. Maybe the scale didn't reflect our efforts but if we let go of our attachment to the number on the scale and look instead to the bigger picture and review our efforts, we can see where we were successful and that success can motivate us to keep going. That's how non-attachment works. So, the next time you are wondering when you will get whatever it is you want, hum a few bars of "Que Sera Sera."

***Today:* Do a mini-meditation before three meals or snacks, eat two meals or snacks mindfully and meditate for fifteen minutes.**

***Today's Journal Question:* What would happen if you let go of your attachment to the number on the scale, on a dress label or a pant size?**

APRIL 8:

DON'T SCRATCH THAT ITCH

If you would like to get better at controlling your impulses, practice with an itch. We all tend to reach for an itchy spot when we feel it. It is almost irresistible. "Almost" being the operative word. You can learn to be with an itch and not scratch it. Here's how. I am sure that sometimes you feel an itch when you are meditating. The next time you do, choose to observe the itch. Study it. Describe it to yourself. Imagine what color it is or shape it takes. Notice as it intensifies and then recedes. Sit with it for as long as you can. If you must scratch, scratch and try again another time. Eventually, you will be able to let it go away on its own. Eventually will be able to avoid acting on it. That is impulse control. This kind of impulse control leads to less emotional eating because if you can sit with an itch and not scratch, you can sit with a feeling and not eat.

***Today:* Do a mini-meditation before three meals or snacks, eat two meals or snacks mindfully and meditate for fifteen minutes.**

***Today's Journal Question:* Try waiting to scratch an itch and write down what it felt like for you to wait the itch out.**

APRIL 9:

COMING BACK FROM THE BRINK

The path to mindful eating is not a straight line. There will be slip ups, setbacks, even full-on binges. Not to worry. You can always begin again. In your dieting days, it is very likely that when you had a slip and "went off your diet," you chastised yourself. Your mind filled with self-loathing thoughts which often led to either quitting the diet altogether or using the slip as an excuse to keep eating until some designated date in the future (usually a Monday). I am happy to tell you that those days are behind you. From now on, if you should slip (defined simply as eating mindlessly) this is what you do:

1. Notice that you slipped.
2. Observe the nature and extent of your slip without judgement (Imagine if a friend is confessing to you. You would hear her out without reprimand, right? Do the same for yourself.)
3. Become curious as to why the slip occurred. Were you tired? Angry? Hurt? Distracted? Bored? Understand the event without rebuke.
4. Offer yourself a compassionate response to why the slip occurred. (Again, it helps to imagine what you would offer a friend and then offer the same loving words to yourself.)
5. Eat your very next meal, or bite, or lick mindfully.

Follow this sequence whenever you find that you stopped eating mindfully. It is a simple remedy, an easy fix.

***Today:* Do a mini-meditation before three meals or snacks, eat two meals or snacks mindfully and meditate for fifteen minutes.**

***Today's Journal Question:* Write down how you can recover from mindless eating.**

APRIL 10:

RIDE THE WAVE

One of the most valuable skills you will achieve as a mindful eater is riding the wave of emotions. If you are a stress eater or an emotional eater of any kind, this skill can change your life! If you have spent time at a beach, you know that waves roll onto the shoreline and then recede. If you are a sail-

or, you know the feel of waves under the boat as they carry you up and down along the water's surface. Drift along with the waves and you are fine. Fight the waves and harm could come. You can view emotions the same way—as waves that come and go. Just like the waves in the oceans all you have to do is float with them.

Observe your emotions objectively and see if you notice this pattern: They come. They crest. They fall. Sometimes in minutes. Other times in hours, but they will follow this pattern. Learn to sit with your emotions without acting on them. Just be present. Notice their ebbs and flows. Pay attention to where you feel them in your body. Watch the thoughts that accompany them. Use your meditation skills to be a curious, impartial spectator of your emotional life. Contrary to what you might think, staying with your emotions causes them to move along more quickly than avoiding or denying them. Evaded emotions linger. They show up again and again in different ways and at different times. Ride the waves of your emotions and then after they've past, acknowledge yourself for not eating over them.

***Today:* Do a mini-meditation before three meals or snacks, eat two meals or snacks mindfully and meditate for fifteen minutes.**

***Today's Journal Question:* Pick an emotion and try to ride its wave and describe the experience as best you can.**

APRIL 11:

I GIVE YOU PERMISSION

The first book I wrote is called *Self-Fullness: The Art of Loving and Caring for Your "Self."* In that book I gave the reader permission to take care of herself without feeling guilty. Repeatedly people have thanked me for giving them that permission because they could not give it to themselves. Having permission to take care of themselves and to put themselves first, liberated them and made them better wives, mothers, sisters, people. I have heard the same about food and eating. A struggle people share is that they feel it is not okay to eat. That it is not okay to love food. They feel like somehow if they were to admit they love food and they gave themselves permission to eat whatever they want, they would eat and eat like there is no tomorrow. They fear gluttony will rule the day. In fact, just the opposite tends to happen.

After an initial free-for-all because they truly don't believe that they can eat whatever they want, people eat less. They find their personal balance between eating and wanting to eat. If you are stuck on your mindful journey because you still don't feel as if it is okay to live the way I am suggesting, I give you permission to do so. I give you permission to love food. I give you permission to end your mindless eating and embrace mindful eating. I give you permission to take care of yourself, to do what is right for you regardless of what others may think, to believe in yourself and to honor all parts of yourself and your body. I give you permission to honor your physical and emotional hungers. I give you permission to buy, prepare and eat the foods that sing to you. I give you permission to trust yourself to do the best you can, when you can without judgment or self-recrimination. I give you permission to be mindful in all you do. I also give you permission to eat 3 meals or snacks mindfully beginning today.

Today: **Do a mini-meditation before three meals or snacks, eat two meals or snacks mindfully and meditate for fifteen minutes.**

Today's Journal Question: **What does it mean to you to have permission to take care of yourself?**

APRIL 12:
GETTING OUT OF A BINGE

So, you've been on your mindful eating journey for a while. You've been meditating some days, but not all. You try to be mindful of your hunger, fullness and taste. As journeys go, you are doing okay. Making some progress. Feeling a little bit better about yourself, your relationship to food and your body—and then you binge. It doesn't occur all at once. It sneaks up on you. A little mindless eating here, a little excess eating there, and before you know you are eating in the same way you did before you started this new approach. No worries. It happens to everyone. Here's what you do: Love yourself. That's right, love yourself. This is no time for self-loathing, bad-mouthing or name-calling. The last thing your binge needs is more fuel to self-sabotage. Instead, love yourself. Binges happen. Now is the time to comfort yourself the way you would a friend who is distressed over a mistake she made. Buy her/yourself flowers. Take her/yourself to a movie. Draw a bath. Get a manicure. Meditate. Do whatever demonstrates self-love to you. Then, begin again. Binges end. Mindless eating ends. All it takes is paying attention on purpose. You can do that. Begin again as many times as you need to. Love yourself as much as you can, whenever you can. You deserve it, even if right now, because you binged, you feel as if you don't.

Today: Do a mini-meditation before three meals or snacks, eat three meals or snacks mindfully and meditate for fifteen minutes.

Today's Journal Question: What is your binge history?

APRIL 13:
WHY DIETS DON'T WORK

Mindful eating is a non-diet approach to weight loss and weight management. I became interested in such an approach after years of my own struggle with weight even though I was "eating right" and years of watching my clients go on and off diets, cycling through the same pounds over and over again. I began researching why diets fail and learned a lot of discouraging facts. For instance, in long-term studies only one in every ten dieters was thinner after five years and four in every ten dieters was heavier. I learned that the body perceives dieting as stressful and releases cortisol, a hormone which causes weight gain. And I also learned that the body has a "defended weight range." This range is unique for each of us and reflects what is biologically healthy for us.

When dieting takes body weight lower than this range, the body reacts by increasing appetite, making food more rewarding to certain parts of the brain, and reducing the number of calories burned, all of which conspire to increase food intake and decrease energy expenditure, bringing the weight back into the defended range. Very discouraging, I know. The research in mindful eating, however, is encouraging. Because mindful eating focuses on internal cues rather than external ones, it is more in tune with the body's weight regulation mechanisms. Dieting pits different brain systems and body regulatory pathways against each other. Mindful eating works in harmony with these systems and puts them in alignment. You may not get the quick weight loss a diet promises but neither will you get the quick rebound weight gain when the diet is over. Mindful eating offers a better long-term strategy than dieting. It may take longer, but the results are more likely to stick.

***Today:* Do a mini-meditation before three meals or snacks, eat three meals or snacks mindfully and meditate for fifteen minutes.**

***Today's Journal Question:* What is your diet history?**

APRIL 14:

I AM SO . . . BORED!

A common reason I hear for why people eat when they are not hungry is that they are bored. "I have nothing else to do," is a frequent refrain. When I ask them what kind of activities they are engaging in, they tell me it doesn't matter. They are bored in exercise class, driving, watching TV, even reading (hopefully you, dear reader, are not!). The kind of boredom they are describing is typically felt when a person is under-stimulated. The moment feels dull or void of fun. At this time their mind wanders to thoughts that reinforce their boredom, such as "this is never going to end" or "how many times do I have to see/do/hear this?" If you find yourself feeling bored (and, by the way, boredom is not only an indication of lack of stimulation but can also be sign of unresolved anger. For more on that check out my book *The Best Diet Begins in Your Mind*), use your mindfulness skills to explore what is going on. Instead of judging your boredom or criticizing your situation, become curious about it. Focus on how boredom feels in your body, where you notice is. Does it change in intensity? What color would you ascribe to it? What shape? Observe your thoughts and rather than attach to them let them float away. By paying attention to your boredom, you will most likely no longer be bored. How's that for a remedy?!

***Today:* Do a mini-meditation before three meals or snacks, eat three meals or snacks mindfully and meditate for fifteen minutes.**

***Today's Journal Question:* What role does boredom play in your eating?**

APRIL 15:

IS MINDFUL EATING TAXING?

In America, today is Tax Day. It's a day when many of us are stressed to the max finishing our tax returns, racing to the post office to meet the midnight deadline, and praying our refund (if we are getting one) comes soon. Taxes are taxing. But is mindful eating taxing, too? Are you finding it difficult, demanding or challenging? If you are, you may be trying too hard. Remember a principle of mindfulness is non-striving. Relax a bit. Give yourself a break. If you remember to eat one bite mindfully you are doing great in my eyes. If you engaged in your meditation practice at least once this week, you are winning. Becoming a mindful eater is a process and it takes a while for it to really take hold. I stumbled about for at least a year before it sank in and became easy. A year.

At first, I was impatient, and then I decided that if mindful eating is going to be my new normal, meaning that it will be with me for the rest of my life, there is no rush to master it. It will come as it comes. I released any need to measure my efforts (i.e., any weight loss or number of minutes I meditated) and simply relaxed into the process. I trusted the research. I trusted my training. I trusted myself to try my best. Today, Tax Day, I offer you the chance to release any stress or strain you are putting on yourself and invite you to trust me, trust this work and most important trust yourself. I invite you to lean into this process and see what happens. Mindful eating does not need to be taxing; it can be pure joy.

***Today:* Do a mini-meditation before three meals or snacks, eat three meals or snacks mindfully and meditate for fifteen minutes.**

***Today's Journal Question:* What taxes you?**

APRIL 16:

THE TEN-MINUTE BREAKFAST

I have a challenge for you. I'd like you to eat your breakfast today slowly—take at least ten minutes. If you are like I was, you eat your breakfast either on the run, in the car, while dressing or quickly over the sink. Even if you do sit down at a table, I suspect you finish your breakfast in under five minutes unless you are doing something else while eating (like reading or answering email). The first time I tried to extend my breakfast to ten minutes I felt tortured. My usual breakfast is yogurt with berries and nuts. That's not a lot of food and ten minutes is a lot of time but I did it. I set a timer for ten minutes and really slowed down. I would take a spoonful and then put the spoon down. I would watch the timer tick down a few seconds before taking my next bite. I paced myself so that I would finish exactly at the ten-minute mark.

As I was clearing my bowl, I noticed something. I felt satisfied and full. I paused for a moment to reflect and realized that by simply slowing down I got more out of my little breakfast than I ever thought I did. This inspired me. When it was time for lunch, I extended my mealtime to fifteen minutes. As I neared the end of the allotted time, I had to really slow down so I wouldn't finish early. I took my last three bites over three minutes—one each minute. Silly I know but when I finished, I felt great. I did it again for dinner. This time I pushed it to thirty minutes. Since that day, I have made it my mission to become a slower eater. I secretly hold contests with friends to see if I can be the last to finish a meal. They don't know I am doing this and I usually win! What I found is that by slowing down, I am more relaxed and naturally more mindful as I eat. I challenge you to try a ten-minute breakfast. What happens for you if you slow down?

***Today:* Do a mini-meditation before three meals or snacks, eat three meals or snacks mindfully and meditate for fifteen minutes.**

***Today's Journal Question:* What happens if you slow down when you eat?**

APRIL 17:
DIETING IS FATTENING

In case you are wondering why in spite of a lifetime of dieting you have still not achieved the weight loss you have been seeking, I have some interesting news. Dieting itself causes weight gain. Diets, even so-called healthy ones, are stressful. The constant vigilance you need to maintain to make sure you are sticking to you causes a stress reaction in the body. And we know that stress puts on weight. The mechanics are quite simple. When our body senses we are under some sort of attack, it reacts with a cascade of hormones designed to give us a fighting chance. One of those hormones that gets triggered in a stress response is cortisol. Cortisol is released during stress to regulate bodily functions including blood sugar levels and blood pressure.

When we are dealing with an acutely stressful situation such as a near-miss while driving, cortisol kicks in to high gear to help with the situation and then returns to normal when the stress is over. When we are under chronic stress, the levels remain high and that is when we get into trouble. An unfortunate side effect of excess cortisol is the accumulation of fat, particularly belly fat. Diets are a form of chronic stress. Day in and day out we are under the demands of the diet. Over time this creates a chronic situation which prevents our cortisol levels from returning to normal and the consequence is excess weight. Mindful eating has the opposite effect. Mindful eating triggers a relaxation response rather than a stress response. In fact, a regular mindful meditation practice reduces stress levels. If you want to lose weight and keep it off, quit dieting and keep going with your mindful eating habits.

***Today:* Do a mini-meditation before three meals or snacks, eat three meals or snacks mindfully and meditate for fifteen minutes.**

Today's Journal Question: **How has dieting made you fat?**

APRIL 18:
YOUR BELLY'S BRAIN

Developing your Inner Wisdom is a key component to becoming a mindful eater. The more you are attuned with your body the better choices you make. Here's some really good news—your body is fully equipped to help you. You have heard of the central nervous system, I am sure. You probably have also heard of the Autonomic Nervous System. But have you ever heard of the Enteric Nervous System (ENS)? Located within the esophagus, stomach and small and long intestines, this nervous system is sometimes referred to as the "belly brain." The ENS is responsible for sensing and controlling your digestive tract. This system communicates with your brain to inform you what, when and how much to eat. When you seek your body's signals for hunger and fullness, when you listen for input on what to eat, and when you feel satisfied, that's your ENS guiding you. Next time you yearn for Inner Wisdom, ask your belly brain. It's right there with ready answers.

Today: **Do a mini-meditation before three meals or snacks, eat three meals or snacks mindfully and meditate for fifteen minutes.**

Today's Journal Question: **What is your reaction to the idea of a "belly brain"?**

APRIL 19:
EATING WITHOUT DISTRACTION—SORT OF

As I am sure you are realizing, becoming a mindful eater is a process. You don't wake up one day a mindful eater. Well, maybe somebody does. I didn't and all of the people I have worked with have not. So, I will assume neither have you. Obviously, the more you practice the easier and more second-natured it becomes. A technique that helped me become a more mindful eater was eating without distractions. Whenever I can, I eat at a table by myself in silence—sort of. My mind is there chattering away so not totally silent. I do, however, set everything aside. No cellphone. No TV. No computer. No iPad. No iPod. No books. No magazines. No mail. You get the picture.

I sit down, take few breaths, do a short mini-meditation to set the mood and then eat. The first few bites are mindful. I savor them enjoying the flavors and aromas, the temperature and texture. Then, slowly without my consent my mind wanders. I start thinking about the clients I will be seeing later in the day or those I already saw. I think about my plans for the weekend or the blog post I want to write.

Before I know it, I am halfway through my meal without tasting another bite. Oops. I could throw my hands up in frustration. Here we go again, eating mindlessly. I could berate myself and chastise myself for trying to "teach this stuff" when I am still mindless. But I don't. I use what just happened to strengthen my mindful eating habits. As soon as I "come to" and recognize what has just occurred, I put my fork (or spoon) down. I take a long deep breath and exhale forcefully. This centers me. I turn my attention to my food (what's left of it anyway) and revisit it as new. I look at its colors and textures. I touch it to feel its temperature. I sniff it to get a whiff of its scent. In other words, I start again. When I am ready, I lift the food to my mouth and begin again. I hang in there mindfully for as long as my mind allows and when I discover my mind has wandered, I catch it and I begin again. I do this over and over again. Some meals this happens only once or twice. Other meals it feels as if this happens every other bite. No worries. Each time I begin again. This is the lesson for today—begin again. Begin as many times as you need to. You cannot begin again too often. Every time you begin again you are strengthening your mindful eating skills. You can do this—again.

***Today:* Do a mini-meditation before three meals or snacks, eat three meals or snacks mindfully and meditate for fifteen minutes.**

***Today's Journal Question:* How does it feel to eat without distractions?**

APRIL 20:
OTHER "COMFORT FOODS"

Many of us seek out "comfort foods" when we are distressed. These foods, usually associated with fond childhood memories, are used to soothe our jagged nerves, mend our broken hearts and cool off our seething anger. They comfort us, hence the name. The desire to comfort ourselves is a natural and healthy one. In psychology circles, we call that "self-soothing." Eating comfort foods in response to a feeling or situation is a form of self-soothing. It can become a problem when eating such foods is our only source of comfort or self-soothing. In addition, there are other unhealthy ways people choose to soothe, including drinking, smoking, and using recreational drugs. Instead, I want you to consider other healthy ways to soothe yourself that are consistent with your efforts to becoming a mindful eater. How about a warm bath? A massage? A meditation session? A conversation with a cherished friend? A cup of herbal tea and a good book? A nap? A swim? A walk with your dog? A cuddle with your cat? Make a list of ten activities you could do when you need some relief from what's happening in your life that does not include food. Keep your list handy so you can refer to it when you need it. Seeking out other ways to comfort yourself is the mindful approach.

***Today:* Do a mini-meditation before three meals or snacks, eat three meals or snacks mindfully and meditate for fifteen minutes.**

***Today's Journal Question:* What else can you do to comfort yourself besides eat?**

APRIL 21:

BUILDING INNER WISDOM

A while back I introduced you to the notion of Inner Wisdom. It may have seemed like a new concept to you at the time but Inner Wisdom has been there for you your whole life. Every day your Inner Wisdom lets you know when you are hungry, thirsty, tired and stressed. You may, however, not be paying attention or choosing to disregard it. Your Inner Wisdom is there when you "have a feeling" about something or someone. Now, with mindful eating, we are bringing your use of Inner Wisdom into the forefront by consciously (mindfully) looking for it. Your Inner Wisdom is guiding you in everything you do, choose to listen. You can build your use of your Inner Wisdom with these simple acts: When you feel the need to go to the bathroom, go! When you feel thirsty, have some water. When you are tired, sleep. When you itch, scratch. When you feel stiff, stretch. When you are hungry, eat. Noticing and acting on these nudges from your Inner Wisdom will strengthen your relationship to it. In time, it will become a vital tool for your overall well-being.

***Today:* Do a mini-meditation before three meals or snacks, eat three meals or snacks mindfully and meditate for fifteen minutes.**

Today's Journal Question: How are you doing with cultivating your Inner Wisdom?

APRIL 22:

KEEPING A FOOD CAUSE–AND-EFFECT DIARY

An effective tool for managing one's weight is keeping a food diary. Keeping a food diary, however, is not an essential part of mindful eating because for some it brings back memories of calorie counting and a focus on quantity over quality. A Food Diary can be a useful tool for mindful eating if you use it a bit differently than you may have in the past. Part of mindful eating is learning what foods work best for your body. In your dieting days, you may have eaten something because it was "allowed" and then had heartburn, gastric distress or fatigue afterwards. Now you can use a Food Diary to understand the effects a food has on you so you can make more mindful choices in the future. To create such a Food Diary, make a chart with six columns. Label the first column FOOD. Label the remaining columns PHYSICAL, MOOD, ENERGY, SLEEP, and BATHROOM.

After you eat (or drink) something, list it in the first column. Then, use the other columns to record what effect the food (or drink) had throughout the day. For example, maybe you had a burrito for lunch and then observed that an hour later you were burping. You would make a note in the PHYSICAL column. Or perhaps you had a latte at 4pm and couldn't fall asleep later that night. Put a comment in the SLEEP column to remember that consequence. Do this for a week (or longer if you prefer) and see what you uncover. Use your discoveries to guide your choices in the future.

Today: **Do a mini-meditation before three meals or snacks, eat three meals or snacks mindfully and meditate for fifteen minutes.**

Today's Journal Question: **If you choose to keep a Food Diary as described above, in what ways do you expect it to help you?**

APRIL 23:

CAN'T STOP EATING? TAKE A WALK

A vital part of mastering mindful eating is learning when your body has had enough food. You learned earlier that we call that Mindful Fullness. An equally vital part, and one which I see people struggle with a lot, is stopping when they are full. Knowing that you are full is half the strategy. The other half is being willing to stop eating. This can be especially hard when you still have food on your plate or when the food you have been eating is a previously "forbidden" food. When your body signals fullness, it is telling you that you have met its nutritional needs. In other words, it is no longer physically hungry. If you eat after this signal you will be eating more food than your body requires and that's what can lead to excess weight. So how do you stop when full if you don't want to?

Here's a tactic I recommend to my clients—take a walk. Move away from the food and take a short walk, maybe ten or fifteen minutes. When you return if you still want to eat the food that remains, eat it. If you don't want to eat it, pack it up and save for another time when you are hungry again. My experience has been that more often than not you won't want to eat after taking the break. Getting up from the table and going for a walk interrupts the automatic (mindless) nature of wanting to keep eating after you know you are full. If you don't want to take a walk, make a phone call, read a few pages in a book, do something. It's the interruption that will lead to success.

***Today:* Do a mini-meditation before three meals or snacks, eat three meals or snacks mindfully and meditate for fifteen minutes.**

***Today's Journal Question:* Besides walking what else could you do when you can't stop eating when you are full?**

APRIL 24:

GASOLINE ON FIRE

I recently read book called *Inner Guru* by Charles D'Angelo. Charles is known as "The Weight Loss Coach," having lost 130 pounds as a teen and making it his life's work to help others do the same. Charles was able to lose his excess weight when he understood the emotional component and addressed it. In his book he remarks, "Eating to heal emotional pain is like putting gasoline on a fire." He is so right! When you add gasoline to a flame it ignites it further, making it harder to extinguish. The fire grows instead of recedes. The same is true when you eat in response to your emotions. Instead of fixing what is wrong you add to the problem. Not only is the underlying problem still there you are now dealing with regret, guilt, self-loathing, and excess weight. Just like finding the right tools to use to put out a fire, find the right tools to deal with your emotions.

Today: Do a mini-meditation before three meals or snacks, eat three meals or snacks mindfully and meditate for fifteen minutes.

T*oday's Journal Question:* What fires might you be stoking with gasoline?

APRIL 25:

IGNITE THE FIRE WITHIN

Since we are speaking of fire, there is a fire I would like you to add gasoline to and that is the fire inside you that drives your desire to heal. When you first began your journey to be a mindful eater, I am sure you were excited. You were motivated and filled with the hope that you have found something that will make a difference in your life. The funny thing about motivation—like fire—if it isn't stoked it will die out. Today I would like you to revisit the reasons you choose to start this journey. If you wrote them down, pull them out. If you didn't, write them now. Think back to when you first heard about mindful eating and what your impressions were. What did you hope to accomplish by taking on this new approach? Did you set any goals for yourself? Did you want lose a specific amount of weight? If yes, why and why that amount? Was your goal to be healthier? More at peace with food? Whatever your reasons keep them in front of you. Review them often. Add to them. Change them. Keep the fire within you lit. It will light the way when things get dark.

***Today:* Do a mini-meditation before three meals or snacks, eat three meals or snacks mindfully and meditate for fifteen minutes.**

Today's Journal Question: What stokes your fire?

APRIL 26:

TASTE SENSATIONS REVISITED

Back in March we explored Mindful Taste and how taste is a key component to mindful eating. It is so important to taste your food. How are you doing with Mindful Taste? Do you taste your food? Or do you eat so fast or with some much distraction that you barely notice? What about what you drink? Are you gulping and slurping or sipping and savoring? The more you can taste the food, the more the food registers with your body and the stronger your body's signals can become to guide you. Keep practicing with taste. In particular pay attention to which foods taste good to you and which don't. If you are eating foods that don't taste good, why are you eating them? Convenience? Habit? Peer pressure? Also, continue to pay attention to how taste changes as you eat and when and if you continue eating in spite of the change. Try to cultivate your inner gourmet and choose the tastiest foods you can find.

***Today:* Do a mini-meditation before three meals or snacks, eat three meals or snacks mindfully and meditate for fifteen minutes.**

***Today's Journal Question:* How have you been surprised by how foods taste?**

APRIL 27:

HEALING SELF-TOUCH

One of the principles of mindfulness that I introduced to you earlier this month was self-compassion. Have you been demonstrating more self-compassion? If you have, good for you! If you are still struggling, I want to share with you a short version of a delightful meditation called Healing Self-Touch which you can do anytime you need to support yourself.

Begin by getting into a comfortable position either seated or lying down and close your eyes. Bring your awareness to your hands and notice what they are touching. Turn your hands so they are face up and take few deep breathes. Imagine your hands are filled with kindness. Gently lift one hand and place it across your body on the other arm. Feel its touch. Next bring your other hand up and place it on your other arm as if you are giving yourself a soft hug. Take a few deep breaths as you gently hold yourself. Stroke your arms lightly if you desire. Feel the comfort and compassion you are offering yourself. Take a few more deep breaths. Stay in this position for as long as feels good for you and when you are ready open your eyes. You can do this short meditation any time you need self-compassion. I encourage you to do it often.

***Today:* Do a mini-meditation before three meals or snacks, eat three meals or snacks mindfully and meditate for fifteen minutes.**

Today's Journal Question: **How can you engage in more self-compassion?**

APRIL 28:

AFTER ALL, TOMORROW IS ANOTHER DAY

One of the nice things about mindful eating is that since there are no rules about what you can and cannot eat, you can eat your favorite foods every day, you just can't eat more of them than your body needs! With mindful eating, one of the habits you are working on is knowing when you are full and when to stop eating. It can be disappointing to stop eating your favorite food when there is some on the plate unless you keep in mind Scarlett O'Hara's famous line from *Gone with the Wind*, "After all, tomorrow is another day." From a mindful eating point of view, that means you can eat what you want again—tomorrow. Or, more specifically, the next time you feel physical hunger.

Today: **Do a mini-meditation before three meals or snacks, eat three meals or snacks mindfully and meditate for fifteen minutes.**

Today's Journal Question: **How might knowing that you can eat your favorite food the next time you are hungry help you stop eating when you are full?**

APRIL 29:

RECOMMIT WHEN YOU FALTER

We all stumble and fall. We all backslide and fail. We all need to start again. I expect, and you should too, that you will make mistakes on your journey to mindful eating. Perhaps the word "mistake" is the wrong word. You will be human and humans go off course. Whenever you notice that you are going off course, recommit. Recommit to this journey. Take a single action to demonstrate to yourself that you would like to get back on track. Recommit by meditating for a few minutes, by eating your next bite mindfully, by paying attention to your sense of fullness, or by journaling about what happened. Be curious. Remind yourself why being a mindful eater is in your best interest. Faltering is not fatal. Quitting is. So simply begin again by recommitting to yourself and this journey.

Today: **Do a mini-meditation before three meals or snacks, eat three meals or snacks mindfully and meditate for fifteen minutes.**

Today's Journal Question: **What can you do to demonstrate your willingness to recommit to this mindful eating journey should you stumble and fall?**

APRIL 30:

REVIEW

If you have been traveling the journey I am setting out for you here, you have been practicing fifteen minutes of daily meditation—most days. If not, that's okay too. One of the principles of mindfulness is non-judgment. No judgment here. What we will do now is take some time to reflect on your experience so far. Here are some questions for you to consider:

1. Have I been consistent with my meditation practice? If yes, how so? If not, what is getting in the way?
2. Have I found a posture that is comfortable for me? What works? What can I try out?
3. Have there been any changes to my eating habits? What changes am I noticing?
4. Have there been any improvements to my sleeping habits or energy levels? If so, what kind of improvements?
5. Can I focus more? Concentrate better?
6. Am I more motivated?
7. Is my life feeling more joyful?
8. Am I enjoying meditation? Why or why not?

Continue practicing at least six times during the week with a goal towards having daily practice.

Today: **Do a mini-meditation before three meals or snacks, eat three meals or snacks mindfully and meditate for fifteen minutes.**

Today's Journal Question: **In what ways has meditating affected your life-and your eating to date?**

MAY

MAY 1:

20-MINUTE MEDITATION AND NOTING

Today you will be adding to your meditation practice in two ways. First, we will be increasing your sitting time to twenty minutes. Second, we will be adding the skill of "noting." Up until now our emphasis has been on breathing. Your practice will remain primarily a breathing practice but today we will expand your experience to include an open awareness concept called "noting." Noting is the practice of briefly labeling what comes into awareness. For example, you are sitting in your practice and your next-door neighbor starts mowing his lawn. The sound of the mower has now come into your awareness. To prevent you from trailing off into a thought stream about the mowing ("Why is he doing that now? I need to mow our lawn! That mower is so loud. He is polluting the air," etc.), you note what is occurring with a label such as "sound" or "noise" and then redirect your practice back to your breath.

The reason to label or note is to interrupt the natural reactive process. It is designed to help you become less reactive to what is going on around you. This is called "non-reactive awareness." When we are less reactive to what is happening to us, we create the time and space to make a more thoughtful choice on how to respond. You put this "non-reactive awareness" into your meditation practice by labeling whatever grabs your attention. It can be a sound, a physical sensation (such as an itch or an ache), a smell, or a thought (such as planning, rehearsing, worrying, etc.). When your awareness is pulled away from your breath, label it and return to the breath. Imagine how this practice can help your eating habits if you learn to pause before reaching for food. To expand your practice to twenty minutes you can use a timer or a guided meditation recording from an app or CD.

Today: **Do a mini-meditation before three meals or snacks, eat three meals or snacks mindfully and meditate for twenty minutes.**

Today's Journal Question: **What kind of thoughts are you prone to noting in your meditation session?**

____

MAY 2:

EAT DESSERT FIRST—A LESSON ABOUT MINDFUL FULLNESS

Today I'd like to explore how fullness can affect your mindful eating experience. If you grew up in a household like I did, dessert was always reserved for after dinner. That meant I would have to eat my entire meal before I was "eligible" for dessert. I understand where my parents were coming from. They were concerned that my sister and I ate "proper meals." Here's the rub—after eating my entire meal I was already full, but I really wanted dessert, so I ate it. Eating dessert after a full meal caused a couple of problems. First, because I was full, the dessert did not taste as good as it would have if I was hungry for it; and second, I now ate more food than my body needed, and I risked gaining weight. A more mindful choice for my parents would have been to offer dessert later when I was hungry again, or, better yet, first! At either time I would have tasted the dessert, enjoyed it more, eaten a portion appropriate for my hunger and gone on my way. Fullness affects taste and taste affects satisfaction. Left unsatisfied you are at danger of eating more because you are "chasing the taste." More on that later.

***Today:* Do a mini-meditation before three meals or snacks, eat three meals or snacks mindfully and meditate for twenty minutes.**

***Today's Journal Question:* When is it easier for you to eat mindfully?**

MAY 3:

PRACTICE NOT PERFECTION

One of the biggest hurdles for me and for many others who try to adopt mindful eating is avoiding their meditation practice. We say we want to practice. We know, and have often experienced, the benefits that come from practicing and yet from time to time (maybe daily even) when it comes time to sit for our practice we resist. This is true even for those who have meditated for years or even decades. Resistance is a natural part of this process. For beginners, a common reason behind the resistance is the thought that we are not "doing it right." Thoughts such as "I can't quiet my mind," or "I can't do this," or "It's too hard" are common refrains. The way I got through these thoughts was by practicing anyway. What I mean is that I sat at my appointed time, turned on the audio (or timer) and waited for it to be over. Or as one of my meditation teachers said, "Fake it 'til you make it!"

Sometimes my mind wandered to my "to-do" list. Other times I made shopping lists or rehearsed a conversation I would have later. There were times when my mind focused on the audio or my breathing. Over time there were more moments like those until eventually I found myself engaged in the meditation. Even today, several years into my practice there are days I have to "fake it" but as long as I am sitting, I am doing my meditation practice. So, if you struggle, resist or avoid, that's okay. No judgment here. Just try to sit. Fake it and you'll eventually make it too!

Today: **: Do a mini-meditation before three meals or snacks, eat three meals or snacks mindfully and meditate for twenty minutes.**

Today's Journal Question: **What can you do to help you deepen your meditation practice?**

MAY 4:
WHAT ARE YOU REALLY HUNGRY FOR?

There are times when we all overeat. Some of those times are planned. Christmas, Thanksgiving and birthdays, perhaps. There are other times when we find ourselves overeating in spite of our best intentions. It is at those times that it becomes valuable to be mindful. Interrupting overeating is a skill that can be learned. Letting go of mindless eating and turning our attention to what is actually going on is the key. My philosophy is that when we are overeating, we are doing so for a very important reason. This excess food or increased feeding is serving some purpose. Mindfulness can help you figure out what that purpose is. When you notice that you are overeating, the question to ask yourself is, "What am I really hungry for?" and then listen for the answer.

To do this, remove yourself from wherever you are eating. Find a comfortable place to sit. Take a few deep breaths. Close your eyes and get centered. Focus your attention on your breath until you feel calm and relaxed, then ask yourself "What am I really hungry for?" Listen for the answer. While you are waiting for your answer to emerge, keep your attention on your breath. When thoughts appear that are not answering the question, acknowledge them and send them on their way. If after a few minutes you sense that no answer is surfacing, that's okay. Stop the meditation and go back to the food, if you still want it. Try asking the question again later. Eventually an answer will emerge. Once you have your answer you can go about addressing it.

For example, let's imagine that the answer to "What am I really hungry for?" showed up as "I am tired and need energy." Great. Now you know that what you need is to restore your energy. How might you do that without eating? Brainstorm solutions such as taking a nap, getting some fresh air, going to sleep earlier, sleeping longer, getting help with a task, or delegating some of your work. Once you arrive at a solution that seems right to you, do it. The more mindful you can be about what you are feeling, the easier it will be to stay the course of mindful eating.

Today: **Do a mini-meditation before three meals or snacks, eat three meals or snacks mindfully and meditate for twenty minutes.**

Today's Journal Question: **What are you really hungry for today?**

MAY 5:

THE POWER OF 10: 10,000, THAT IS.

Mindfully incorporating exercise into your life is another part of mindful eating. Exercise, as a part of Outer Guidance, is used to enhance your body's health and your emotional well-being, not to facilitate weight loss. In my TAME Your Appetite Programs, we use walking as the exercise of choice. We use walking because for most people it is a form of exercise that is relatively easy to add to one's life. A good pair of walking shoes and a sidewalk are pretty much all you need. Walking is truly a wonderful form of exercise and one that I have embraced since college. I enjoy walking so much that I have walked three full marathons (a marathon is 26.2 miles), four half marathons and countless 3Ks, 5Ks and 10Ks. If you already walk for exercise, you may know that experts recommend that we take 10,000 steps each day for optimal health. If you are not walking for exercise, I would highly recommend it.

In my TAME programs, participants use a pedometer or other form of step counter to measure their number of daily steps. We start wherever each person is and slowly add steps in accordance with how each body responds. There is no race or contest involved, just mindful awareness of the body's response to gentle exercise. You don't have to be a participant in a TAME program to use walking as a tool for Outer Guidance. You can begin right now, on your own.

Here's what you do: (1) Get a good pair of walking shoes and the right kind of socks. Any reputable sporting goods store should be able to hook you up. (2) Find an app on your iPhone or purchase a fitness tracker and set up it up to count your steps. (3) Count your steps for one week, making no effort to add extra steps. Just do what you normally do. We are getting baseline. (4) At the end of the week, calculate your daily average number of steps. (5) Set a goal to walk 10% more the next week. This means if you currently average 1,000 steps a day, shoot for 1,100 steps the following week. You can add steps simply by taking stairs instead of elevators, parking a bit farther away from your destination, walking to do errands and taking the dog out more often. 6) Continue to increase your daily step count at a pace that feels right for you working towards the magic goal of 10,000 steps. In TAME, we use 10% increases as a starting point but that is an arbitrary number; use what works best for you. Pay attention to how your body feels, your energy levels, your sleep patterns and your mood. If you are tired or run down, walk less. If you feel great, walk some more. (7) If you want to be deliberate about your walking, identify a safe place in your neighborhood to walk (for example a park, walking path, or shopping mall) and make a daily walk a habit. Find a friend to walk with to make it more fun or simply enjoy the time you have to be by yourself. Regardless of how many steps you take or how far you go, remain mindful of your body and it feels before, during and after your walk.

***Today:* Do a mini-meditation before three meals or snacks, eat three meals or snacks mindfully and meditate for twenty minutes.**

***Today's Journal Question:* What are your thoughts about walking as a tool for health and well-being but not for weight loss?**

MAY 6:
TRUST WITH FOOD

Do people trust you? Do they trust that you will show up when you say you will? Do they trust you that you will do what you say you will do? Do they trust you with their children, their pets, their secrets? Do you trust you? Do you trust that if you say you are going to do something, you will do it? Do you trust yourself around food? Many who struggle with diet and weight issues feel untrustworthy. How many times have you said, "I will never eat raw cookie dough again," only to succumb the next time you have a bad day? Or how many diets have you started on a Monday only to fall off by Wednesday? When we fall back on our word, we damage our self-esteem. We lose faith in ourselves and our ability to change.

I want to help you build trust in yourself. I want you to be able to go anywhere and KNOW that you will be at peace with food. The more you practice mindful eating techniques, the more you sit for your daily meditation practice, the more second nature mindful eating becomes. You don't have to be perfect, just consistent. With consistency your confidence in yourself as a mindful eater will grow and you will be able to trust that regardless of the situation you will act in your own best interest and make mindful choices.

***Today:* Do a mini-meditation before three meals or snacks, eat three meals or snacks mindfully and meditate for twenty minutes.**

***Today's Journal Question:* How trustworthy are you?**

MAY 7:

MINDFUL MOVEMENT

There are many types of meditations and many ways to meditate. The mindfulness-based meditation we use as a basis of mindful eating is one type. Others include: Zen, Vipassana, Metta, Hindu and Transcendental. I encourage you to do a little Googling and learn about these. You may find one you really like. These meditations are all done in a seated position but there are also moving meditations. These are types of meditations have moving your body as the focus of your attention and can be a wonderful addition to a sitting meditation practice. Moving meditations include walking, yoga, Qi Gong, and Tai Chi. You can find classes teaching these forms of meditation at YMCAs, yoga studios, recreation centers and online. Search these out and have some fun. All of them help you get in touch with your body and your mind.

***Today:* Do a mini-meditation before three meals or snacks, eat three meals or snacks mindfully and meditate for twenty minutes.**

***Today's Journal Question:* What kind of mindful movement can you add to your life?**

MAY 8:

CROWDING OUT

If you are finding you are having a hard time giving up old habits, you are not alone. Research tells us that once a habit is entrenched in your psyche it really can't be removed, but it can be overwritten. It works the way old video and cassette tapes work, if you remember those. In the old days, if you recorded something on a tape you could record over it. The old recording is still on the tape but you don't see or hear it anymore. You only hear the new recording. Our brain's neural pathways work in the same way. Scientists tell us that the way to create a new habit is to "crowd out" an old one. What does it mean to "crowd out" an old habit? Simply, you repeat a new habit so often that the old habit recedes into the background. I use this technique when I am helping people develop healthier eating habits.

Rather than tell them never to eat sugar again, I encourage them to add one fruit a day until eating a single fruit feels like a habit. Then we add a second fruit or a salad. As they practice this, they slowly replace their sugar-filled foods with healthier versions with little or no effort. You can use "crowding out" to help change other habits too. Let's say you watch too much TV and all that TV leads to mindless eating. To ask you to quit watching TV is a useless request, especially if you are a die-hard Games of Thrones fan. Instead, find another habit you would like to develop and use it to "crowd out" the TV. For example, use exercise. Add a half hour walk to your daily routine. That will be thirty minutes a day when you are not watching TV. It's that simple. Begin today.

***Today:* Do a mini-meditation before three meals or snacks, eat three meals or snacks mindfully and meditate for twenty minutes.**

***Today's Journal Question:* What bad habit can you crowd out?**

MAY 9:
WILLPOWER WON'T CUT IT

Social psychologist Roy F. Baumeister has been studying willpower for years. Among his findings is that people have a lot of desires and, no surprise, eating was the most frequently reported desire. Dr. Baumeister also found that willpower and our ability to make decisions is subject to fatigue. What this means is that the more decisions we have to make, or the more times we have to exercise our "willpower," the less we have of it as the day goes by. We actually get tired of making decisions so that by the end of the day or at the end of a particularly difficult time in our lives, we no longer have the physical or mental capability to make well-informed decisions or take the correct action and we give into the easiest choice. In other words, we give into temptation.

Trying to heal food issues with willpower won't work. If the answer lies not with willpower, where does it lie? It lies with your environment and overall lifestyle. Set yourself up for success by mastering the tools that support your new choice to be a mindful eater. Mindful eating does not demand willpower. All it asks for is your attention. Think about all the food-related decisions you have to make in a day. It can be a constant struggle. When you can rely on your Inner Wisdom and Outer Guidance to choose your food, you don't have to rely on willpower. Willpower becomes part of the process when you are trying to obey the artificial sanctions of a diet. Decision-making about what to eat becomes a chore when you are not tuned into your body and its needs. Practice your daily meditations and mini-meditations. Check in with your Inner Wisdom regularly. Incorporate Outer Guidance. Eat without distractions. Savor your foods. And when you do, you will not need willpower. You will not suffer from willpower fatigue.

***Today:* Do a mini-meditation before three meals or snacks, eat three meals or snacks mindfully and meditate for twenty minutes.**

***Today's Journal Question:* What role has willpower fatigue played in your life?**

MAY 10:

A MINDFUL ENVIRONMENT

We live in a world where food is ubiquitous. Social scientists have a name for it. They call it "the obesogenic environment." Living in an obesogenic environment means living in a world that promotes weight gain and contributes to obesity. Included in this definition is how easy it is to get food. Unlike a few generations ago, food is available twenty-four hours a day, seven days a week everywhere. It means that our food products are so laden with fats and sugars that we can gain weight eating the same kind of food our ancestors ate, only ours is in poorer, unhealthier forms. And it refers to the sedentary nature of our culture that requires very little physical effort to get tasks done. Trying to lose weight, or even maintain weight, in such a setting can be difficult unless you set yourself up for success. One way to do that is to mindfully set up your environment to foster health and well-being.

Think about the environments to which you are exposed. Your home, car, work, school, house of worship, neighborhood, etc. Of these environments, which one (or ones) could you exert some influence over with regard to food, health and well-being? For me, the environments I can control included my kitchen, my office and my car. In support of my mindful eating efforts, I organized each of these spaces to reflect my new habits. In my kitchen, I make sure that the only food on the counters are fruits and vegetables. Everything else found at home are in a cabinet or pantry. I have some "rules"—no eating in my office or car. When it is time to eat during work hours, I go to the office kitchen. I take food from home so I could enjoy what I wanted and not choose whatever co-workers might have left sitting on the counter. If I get hungry while driving, I pull over to eat. If I am traveling a long distance, I bring my own food. These efforts may not seem like a lot but they were constant reminders of my commitment to mindful eating.

***Today:* Do a mini-meditation before three meals or snacks, eat three meals or snacks mindfully and meditate for twenty minutes.**

***Today's Journal Question:* What can you do to shape your environment in support of your goals?**

MAY 11:
I'M NOT A SKINNY MINNIE EITHER

People who meet me for the first time are surprised (maybe disappointed) that I am not a skinny-minnie. I come from a long line of strong German women who are a bit thicker and sturdier than I might prefer. I have always been this way. I have a picture of myself at age two years old and when I look at it, I marvel at how I have the same body shape now as I did then. I can exercise and diet until the cows come home and I will never reshape my body into a five-foot-seven thin-boned specimen like my sister (who takes after our father's side of the family).

Nature is what nature is. What I have learned is that you don't have to be thin to be healthy, or beautiful or loveable. What is most important is being the best version of you that there can be. Becoming a mindful eater has taken me to where I need to be. Would I like to be a few pounds lighter, sure, maybe, I don't know? Would I give up my health, peace of mind and over all well-being to drop some weight? No way! As you continue your journey to mindful eating, keep in mind what you would like to achieve and measure that alongside who you really are. My guess is that when you do that you will find that you are closer than you think you are.

***Today:* Do a mini-meditation before three meals or snacks, eat three meals or snacks mindfully and meditate for twenty minutes.**

***Today's Journal Question:* How close are you to whom or what you want to be?**

MAY 12:

YOU DON'T HAVE TO BE PERFECT

Have you heard of the 80/20 rule? In business circles, it is known as The Pareto Principle. This principle states that 80% of results come from 20% of efforts. I apply this rule to mindful eating and say, "You don't have to be perfect to achieve success." I offer this to you because so many of my clients complain that because they can't (or don't) eat mindfully all the time so they believe they are failing. Nothing could be farther from the truth. If you eat mindfully 20% of the time you are heads above the rest of humanity who eats mindlessly 99% of the time (That's my guess. I don't have an actual figure, but it feels right to me.) What I am trying to convey to you is to give yourself credit for what you are doing and leave the rest behind. Keep your goal of becoming a mindful eater in front of you and do your best. If 20% of your meals and snacks are mindful by now, you are a rock star. Keep it going! They only way to truly fail is to quit.

***Today:* Do a mini-meditation before three meals or snacks, eat three meals or snacks mindfully and meditate for twenty minutes.**

***Today's Journal Question:* In what ways has perfectionism been an issue for you?**

MAY 13:

THE MINDFUL CARROT

Today I'd like you to do something fun. Okay, maybe silly or unusual. But, with the right spirit and intention, it can be fun. I want you to mindfully engage a carrot. Begin by going to your local market and buying the most beautiful, vibrant organic carrot you can find. Bring the carrot home and with love and adventure in your heart, place it on your kitchen counter. Assemble a cutting board, a sharp knife, some paper towels and a bowl. Take your carrot and with full attention, wash it. Feel the water as it rains upon the carrot. Notice how the carrot top wilts as it gets moist. Gently wash the carrot with your fingers and feel the texture against your skin. What does it feel like? Smooth? Crinkly? Gritty? Next, pat the carrot dry with the paper towels and when you are done hold the carrot in your palms for a moment. Acknowledge the carrot. Acknowledge the farmers who grew it and the merchants who sold it. Thank them all, silently or aloud. Now admire the carrot. Its color and size. Look at the carrot as if you have never seen one before. If you had to describe it to a friend, how would you describe it?

When you are ready, place the carrot on the cutting board and pick up the knife. Slowly and deliberately begin to peel or cut the carrot. Whichever you prefer. If you choose to peel it, save the slivers you slice off. Sniff them and play with them before tossing them aside. Then slowly and methodically, cut the carrot anyway you like. Slice it into small circles. Carve it into match sticks. Dice it into tiny pieces. Take your time. Notice if any juice oozes from the carrot. Does its aroma reach your nose? Are your fingers turning orange? When you have finished slicing and dicing, take a step back and look again at the carrot. See it now in its different form. Run your fingers through the pieces. Pick one up and study it. Spend time with your carrot. When you are ready, put your carrot pieces into a bowl. Plan to eat them as part of a meal or snack the next time you feel hungry. When you eat the carrot, observe if it tastes different because of the loving care you put into washing and slicing it. I think it may end up being the most delicious carrot you've ever tasted.

***Today:* Do a mini-meditation before three meals or snacks, eat three meals or snacks mindfully and meditate for twenty minutes.**

***Today's Journal Question:* Reflect on your experience of preparing and eating a carrot mindfully.**

MAY 14:

MINDFUL NATURE

What kind of nature is near you? The ocean? A lake, stream or pond? A park? The beach? A garden? Spend some time in nature today to enhance your mindfulness. Pick a location and when you are there engage all your senses. What do you see? What do you smell? What can you touch? What do you hear? How do you feel? How can being in touch with nature help with your mindful eating? Use your journal to explore these questions. My time in nature is typically a walk near the beach. I am lucky to be in Southern California where the weather is beautiful almost every day. My favorite thing to do is start my day with a walk near the Santa Monica Pier. The fresh air, blue sky, peaceful surf and squawking seagulls calm me. After my walk, I feel more centered, clearer and more focused. The days I am able to take such a walk are usually more pleasant for me than the rest. It is easier for me to remain mindful about my eating when my mind is still. What about you?

***Today:* Do a mini-meditation before three meals or snacks, eat three meals or snacks mindfully and meditate for twenty minutes.**

***Today's Journal Question:* How can time in nature assist with your mindful eating goals?**

MAY 15:

MINDFUL CHOICES

Over the weeks and months that you and I have been on this journey I have used the phrase "mindful choices." Let's explore what mindful choices mean. Primarily when I speak of mindful choices, I am referring to food choices made using both your Inner Wisdom and Outer Guidance. First, when you combine both of these aspects of mindful eating you arrive at decisions that meet your nutritional and weight loss needs. Mindful choices also refer to the behavioral choices you make when you pay full attention to a situation. For example, you are tired and you decide to go to sleep early rather than watch late-night TV. In this example, you are paying attention to your body's needs and honoring it. Finally, mindful choices mean knowingly choosing a different response to an emotion. For example, if you choose to go for a run after an argument with your neighbor rather than rip open bag of pretzels, you have made a mindful choice. Simply stated, mindful choices are choices made with your full attention and awareness. They are the essence of mindful living.

***Today:* Do a mini-meditation before three meals or snacks, eat three meals or snacks mindfully and meditate for twenty minutes.**

***Today's Journal Question:* What mindful choices did you make today?**

MAY 16:

MINDFUL DAY OF BEAUTY

Regardless of what you weigh, regardless of where you are in your journey to mindful eating, regardless of how old you are, it is important to appreciate your own unique beauty. Today is the day to do that. Today is the day to get a manicure, get a pedicure, have a massage, get a facial, shave your legs, tweeze your brows, get new makeup, cut your hair, curl your hair, straighten your hair. Today is the day to appreciate yourself and to give yourself some extra special attention.

***Today:* Do a mini-meditation before three meals or snacks, eat three meals or snacks mindfully and meditate for twenty minutes.**

***Today's Journal Question:* What does beauty mean to you?**

MAY 17:

A TOUGH DAY TIP

If you are having a tough day, ask yourself this simple question: What would I do if I felt better? Then do it.

***Today:* Do a mini-meditation before three meals or snacks, eat three meals or snacks mindfully and meditate for twenty minutes.**

***Today's Journal Question:* Describe what you did to feel better today.**

MAY 18:

A KINDER, MORE PATIENT YOU

Did you kick yourself today? I don't mean literally a bump to the shin, but did you knock yourself today? Put yourself down? Criticize yourself for any reason? Call yourself "stupid" or "idiot"? I hope not, but if you did let's take a moment to discuss such actions. If you were raised in a tough love family, being criticized or judged may have been your family's style of communication or motivation. If it was, it was most likely because your parents were raised the same way. That's all they knew. It is also possible you think that condemning yourself is the only way to get you to do something.

Having worked with people for over two decades I have observed that self-kindness is more effective than self-criticism in making sustainable change. Sure, you can force yourself to do something, but it is unlikely that something will be a permanent change. You wouldn't kick a puppy to teach it to sit, why kick yourself? Remember, trying to change a lifetime of poor habits will take time. During this transition I want to suggest that you be kinder and more patient with yourself than you have ever before. Cuddle the puppy, don't strike her. Wrap yourself in love and support instead of disapproval and rejection.

Today: **Do a mini-meditation before three meals or snacks, eat three meals or snacks mindfully and meditate for twenty minutes.**

Today's Journal Question: **How can you be kinder and more patient with yourself today?**

MAY 19:

CONSCIOUS AND DELIBERATE ACTION

Do you remember Aesop's Fable of the tortoise and the hare? In that fable the tortoise and the hare run a race. The hare, being arrogant and overconfident and convinced he will win the race, stops in the middle to nap. When he awakens, he discovers that the tortoise, who had been slowly and consistently plodding along, had crossed the finish line first. When we stop and start the actions needed to win our race (whether it is weight loss, saving money or getting a new job, you name it) we are much like the hare, so sure we will get there we feel we don't have to put in much effort. What I have learned is that consistent and deliberate action gets us where we want to go. Transferring $50 a week into a savings account has you saving $2,600 a year. Sending out a resume a day will get you that new job. And practicing mindful eating every day will change your relationship with food forever.

Today: **Do a mini-meditation before three meals or snacks, eat three meals or snacks mindfully and meditate for twenty minutes.**

Today's Journal Question: **What conscious deliberate actions can you take today and every day?**

MAY 20:

STOP A BINGE WITH MINDFULNESS

Being trapped inside a binge is a distressing situation. Feeling as if you have no control to stop mindless eating leaves you feeling helpless and defeated. Whether your overeating lasts an evening or a few weeks you can get out of it. All you need to do is choose to be mindful. Just noticing what you are doing breaks the spell. You can keep eating but pay attention as you do. You can even verbally express what is happening. "Now I am putting yet another piece of pizza in my mouth." "I am still shoveling in the chips without stopping." "I am running to the store to buy more comfort food." Whatever you are doing, notice it, acknowledge it, label it. Observe it like a sociologist studying another culture—with detachment. No judgment. Just objectivity. Berating yourself is unlikely to get the binge to stop sooner, but noticing it can. Just stop for a moment, notice what you are doing and breathe. You can go back to your food after the breaths. Keep noticing what you are doing and pausing for breaths and you will find the binge slowing down and eventually stopping.

Today: **Do a mini-meditation before three meals or snacks, eat three meals or snacks mindfully and meditate for twenty minutes.**

Today's Journal Question: **Next time you find yourself mindlessly eating or in a binge, what will you do to help yourself stop?**

MAY 21:

REMINDER—WHY DID YOU COME ON THIS JOURNEY TO MINDFUL EATING?

We are in your fifth month of mindful eating and now might be a good time to revisit your reasons for starting this journey in the first place. Reminding ourselves of why we started a new venture and what we are gaining from it can keep us going, especially during the rough patches. If you are like most people who find their way here, you probably came to mindful eating looking to lose weight. What you had been doing wasn't working and you were looking for a new way. The non-diet approach may have been appealing so you decided to give it a shot.

That is great reason to come on board. Was there anything else? Did you come for any other reasons? Were you looking for a different relationship with food? A new way to handle your emotions? A better way of living? If you weren't, have you since discovered that mindful eating can do more for you than help you lose weight? Think about your reasons for being here and what new reasons you may have to stay the course. We all lose our motivation from time to time and second-guess our decisions to do something new. Remembering our reasons for starting can help us stay on track.

***Today:* Do a mini-meditation before three meals or snacks, eat three meals or snacks mindfully and meditate for twenty minutes.**

***Today's Journal Question:* Write down why you came on this journey to mindful eating as reminder to yourself for those days when you may want to throw it all away.**

MAY 22:

BROKEN TOOLS WON'T FIX WHAT IS BROKEN

The other day my toilet broke. Nothing serious, just needed a new handle. I had done this type of repair before on a different toilet so I knew how to fix it. I took a quick ride to my local hardware store and purchased the replacement part. When I got home, I got to work. I took apart the broken handle and went install the replacement when I noticed that the wrench I needed to use was broken. Can't fix a broken handle with a broken wrench. This incident got me thinking. We can't fix anything with broken tools, especially ourselves.

When we try to fix what is wrong with us with programs, suggestions and processes that don't work, we get nowhere. Trying to fix something broken with broken tools won't work. We need better tools. Mindful eating and mindfulness are those better tools. By now I hope you are experiencing the benefits that mindful eating and mindfulness have on your weight, your self-esteem and your life in general. The tools offered here (Inner Wisdom, Outer Guidance, meditation) function beautifully. They are tools that you can count on. They will never break.

***Today:* Do a mini-meditation before three meals or snacks, eat three meals or snacks mindfully and meditate for twenty minutes.**

***Today's Journal Question:* What broken tools are you still using?**

MAY 23:

FORGIVENESS

Alexander Pope, the 18th century poet, famously said, "To err is human; to forgive, divine." I have a question for you: how forgiving are you? Do you forgive easily—bygones being bygones—or do you hold grudges? Can you forgive some transgressions and not others? Can you forgive yourself? If you look up the definition of forgiveness in the Merriam-Webster dictionary, you will see that it defines forgiveness as the giving up of a resentment or a claim for compensation. I often define it as releasing a debt. Forgiveness is not acceptance or approval. It is a state of mind wherein you stop punishing the transgressor for whatever she or he may have done. This includes you. When you forgive, you release yourself from the hold that offense has over you. You release yourself.

Sometimes we hear stories of victims of crime who forgive their assailant. You may wonder why. When interviewed, these people consistently say they forgive so they can move on and not be burdened by the events of the past. Whom do you need to forgive? Do you need to forgive yourself? As you go through your day today, forgive those who do you wrong. Forgive the driver who cut you off on the highway. Forgive your doctor who is running late for your appointment. Forgive yourself if you ate or acted mindlessly. See how forgiveness makes you feel. Then, when you are ready, forgive those who have truly wronged you, including yourself.

***Today:* Do a mini-meditation before three meals or snacks, eat three meals or snacks mindfully and meditate for twenty minutes.**

***Today's Journal Question:* Write yourself a letter of forgiveness for something you have done that is getting in the way of your moving forward.**

MAY 24:

MORE ON EMOTIONAL EATING

Emotional eating, or what some people call stress eating, explains a lot of the excess weight people carry. Being mindful of your emotions and how you respond to them is a core skill in becoming a mindful eater. Remember mindful eating means eating in response to physical hunger, not emotional hunger. A tool I use in helping people break the automatic reach for food when they feel an emotion is called, "Drop and Give Me Ten." The method behind this tool is simple—when the urge to eat in response to an emotion hits, stop what up are doing and before you open the fridge, bag or carton, sit down. Right there, where you are, sit. On a chair or on the floor. Sit and take ten deep breaths.

After you have completed the ten breaths you can go back to the food you were about to eat or you can choose to do something different. "Drop and Give Me Ten" works to interrupt the mindless move towards food. The pause it creates gives you space to think about what else you can do besides eat. Sometimes you will choose to eat and if you do you will be eating with full knowledge and intention, in other words mindfully. Other times, the pause will stop you from eating and allow you to pursue a different way to cope with your feelings.

***Today:* Do a mini-meditation before three meals or snacks, eat three meals or snacks mindfully and meditate for twenty minutes.**

***Today's Journal Question:* Try "Drop and Give Me Ten" and then write about how it felt to create a pause between your emotion and your actions.**

MAY 25:
PAY APPRECIATION FORWARD

I love what I do. When I was a lawyer, not so much! But these days in my work as a psychologist and mindful eating instructor, I like what I do. Knowing that I help people grow, meet goals, lose weight, feel better about themselves makes the long hours worthwhile. I don't do what I do to win awards or get acknowledgments, but when a client thanks me for my help it sure makes my day. Just this morning a clinical patient who has been having a particularly difficult time called me to say thank you. She wanted me to know that she appreciates me and all I do for her and others. Her call really touched me. I know being able to say what she said made her feel good too. Telling people we appreciate them is a wonderful gift for them and for you. Is there someone who is making a difference in your life? Someone whose efforts you might be taking for granted? What about the dry cleaner who always greets you with a smile and a joke? Or the barista who gets your order right each time? Today let someone know you appreciate them. You can call, email, text or visit. Notice how you feel after you make this gesture. Does how you feel affect your food and eating choices today?

***Today:* Do a mini-meditation before three meals or snacks, eat three meals or snacks mindfully and meditate for twenty minutes.**

***Today's Journal Question:* Whom can you show appreciation for and why?**

MAY 26:
SIZE MATTERS

As you become more attuned to your Inner Wisdom you will be able to read your body and know what, when and how much food you need. This means you will measure your Mindful Hunger and Mindful Fullness before, during and after your meal or snack. These hunger and fullness cues will guide you in your eating. You will notice that your levels of hunger and fullness, as well as the foods that will meet your needs, will vary day by day, even minute by minute. Sometimes you will need more food, other times less. Sometimes you will need heavy, hearty food, other times light and fresh will fit the bill. In addition, some foods will fill you up and keep you satisfied longer than others. Stay aware to how different size meals and different types of food affect your energy level, physical needs, and body's satiety. Notice when you need more food, when you need less. All of these insights cultivate your Inner Wisdom and become the new roadmap for your weight management goals.

***Today:* Do a mini-meditation before three meals or snacks, eat three meals or snacks mindfully and meditate for twenty minutes.**

***Today's Journal Question:* Document what you learn about the roles that hunger, fullness and quantity play in your eating habits.**

MAY 27:
ACTIVE SELF-CARE

Self-care. It means different things to different people. I use the words "self-care" to mean those actions we take that support our physical and emotional health. Self-care actions can be daily tasks, weekly activities or even monthly events. For me, my daily self-care includes: getting into bed by 10 or 10:30 most nights; showering; brushing and flossing my teeth; meditating; writing in my gratitude journal; and eating healthfully. Other self-care activities I engage in are getting manicures and pedicures; having my eyebrows shaped; going to the gym; drinking plenty of water; reading a good book; setting boundaries around receiving and responding to phone calls, emails, and texts; and spending time with family and friends. Self-care can also include massages, acupuncture, doctor appointments, therapy, vacations, and even moisturizers. The thing about self-care is that it usually needs to be arranged, prioritized, and executed. It is so easy to get swept up in "life" that we forget to take care of ourselves. Self-care is an essential component of mindful eating because it encourages us to pay attention to ourselves and our needs, and paying attention is the essence of mindfulness.

What do you do to take care of yourself? Is self-care a priority or do you fall to the bottom of your daily "To-Do" list? Beginning today, pick one self-care action that you are willing to do on a regular basis and schedule it. If your action affects others (for example, you want to go for a weekly massage and that means you need someone to watch the kids), let them know. Explain that your self-care is important for your well-being and that when you are at your best, you are at your best for them too. If you are concerned that taking care of yourself is selfish or you are not sure where to start, take a look at my book *Self-Fullness: The Art of Loving and Caring for Your Self.* It is devoted to making self-care acceptable.

Today: **Do a mini-meditation before three meals or snacks, eat three meals or snacks mindfully and meditate for twenty minutes.**

Today's Journal Question: **What self-care actions do you do and which ones would you like to add to your routine?**

MAY 28:

RELAX FOR MORE FOCUS

Do you know what palming is? It's a technique used to relax the eyes. Derived from the Bates Method for visual improvement, to palm, you close your eyes and rest palms of your hands on your eyes, blocking out all light and hold there for a minute or two, longer if you like. Hold gently, do not put pressure on your eyeballs. When you remove your palms, your eyes are more relaxed and if you are like me, you have a bit better focus. You can repeat the palming technique as often as you like. I do it whenever my eyes feel tired. What happens for our eyes with palming can happen for our minds with relaxing. Relaxation facilitates focus. Whether it is literal visual focus or enhanced concentration, relaxing does the body and mind good. Spend a few minutes each day relaxing. Find a quiet space and unwind. You don't need to do anything special, just be. If it helps, take a few deep breaths and close your eyes. When you're done, see if you, too, feel more focused and attentive.

Today: **Do a mini-meditation before three meals or snacks, eat three meals or snacks mindfully and meditate for twenty minutes.**

***Today's Journal Question:* Relax for five minutes today and reflect on what happened.**

MAY 29:

MINDFUL READING

There is nothing better than a good book. Well, maybe some things are better, but a good book ranks pretty high. Personally, I love to read non-fiction, especially books related to my fields of interest—psychology, mindfulness, and nutrition. I encourage you to do some reading in these fields too while you are on this journey with me. A few minutes or pages a day of "contemplative reading" is a wonderful way to enhance your progress. You may be wondering what to read. There are so many outstanding authors to choose from. Here are some authors who write about mindfulness and mindful eating you might like to check out: Elisha Goldstein, Jon Kabat-Zinn, Jack Kornfield, Jean Kristeller, Andrea Lieberstein, Thich Nat Hahn, Kristen Neff, Lynn Rossy, and Sharon Salzburg. Consider assembling a few friends to form a book club and read these books together.

***Today:* Do a mini-meditation before three meals or snacks, eat three meals or snacks mindfully and meditate for twenty minutes.**

***Today's Journal Question:* Pick a book, read a few minutes a day and write about how what you reading influences your mindful eating journey.**

MAY 30:

BUILD A COMMUNITY

Changing habits is hard. Hopefully having me along is helping you. Yesterday I suggested you gather some friends together and form a book club to read mindfulness and mindful eating books together. One reason I made that recommendation is that community helps facilitate change, especially a community of like-minded people. If you have been traveling this mindful eating journey alone, think about inviting someone to join you. If you don't want to do that, find a meditation group or mindfulness classes and connect with people there. Explore Meetup.com groups for ideas. You can also join my community through my newsletter and social media platforms. However, you choose to go about it, find like-minded people to share your journey. You will get support, knowledge and insight you can't get on your own.

***Today:* Do a mini-meditation before three meals or snacks, eat three meals or snacks mindfully and meditate for twenty minutes.**

***Today's Journal Question:* Where could you find like-minded people to share you journey with?**

MAY 31:

HOW TO BINGE MINDFULLY

At this point in your journey, you are most likely eating mindfully more often than not. That's great news. You may also be still overeating or bingeing, much to your chagrin. That is also okay. Remember this journey is a process, not a straight line. Binges will happen. One way to decrease their frequency is to increase your meditation practice, especially the mini-meditations before your meals and snacks. The research investigating mindfulness-based eating supports this approach. Another way to decrease your bingeing is to binge mindfully. What? When you binge, do so with full awareness of what you are doing. If you are going to binge, give yourself permission to do so.

Acknowledge that in this moment this is your way to deal with your life. Sit at the table. Choose the most delicious desirable food you can think of. Put the food onto pretty plates and bowls. Use your best silver and crystal. Play soothing music and light some candles. Seriously. Giving your binge as much attention as you give to a meal or snack will reduce the binge. You will naturally slow down, naturally eat less and naturally feel full sooner.

***Today:* Do a mini-meditation before three meals or snacks, eat three meals or snacks mindfully and meditate for twenty minutes.**

***Today's Journal Question:* Describe your last binge and how you could have done it mindfully.**

JUNE

JUNE 1:

THE 25-MINUTE BUMP

It's time to bump up your meditation practice again. This time to twenty-five minutes. If you feel ready to extend your sitting time, set your timer for twenty-five minutes and go for it. Many people tell me that going up to twenty-five minutes makes a big difference in their practice. They report fewer chattering thoughts and more focus on the object of their attention.

Remember, if you are not ready for this bump, no worries. That's just fine. Pat yourself on the back for what you have done so far. If you are still not doing any meditation at all, reflect on what is holding you back. What is your resistance? Fear? Uncertainty? Self-consciousness? Whatever maybe getting in your way is worthy of investigation. Be curious about your resistance. What is it trying to tell you? What can you learn from it? Be kind to yourself. Examine what is going on from a stance of non-judgment and self-compassion. If you are really struggling, consider those meditation classes I mentioned earlier. Check one out. Sitting with others can be very inspiring. Continue practicing at least six times a week keeping track in your journal or log.

***Today:* Do a mini-meditation before three meals or snacks, eat three meals or snacks mindfully and meditate for twenty-five minutes.**

***Today's Journal Question:* How does it feel to have a twenty-five-minute-a-day meditation practice?**

JUNE 2:

ENJOY A BUFFET

Once a month I join some friends at a local salad bar buffet-style restaurant for lunch. I enjoy seeing these friends and look forward to each outing. This restaurant is designed so that as soon as you walk in you are at the front of the buffet line. You take a tray and a plate and walk along the buffet piling on one food item after another until you arrive at the cashier. After paying, you enter the rest of the restaurant which has several more stations filed with soups, pastas, entrees, breads and desserts. What a feast! Before I became mindful, I would do as the others did and pile my plate up high with whatever I saw as I moved along the buffet line to the cashier (sure it was salad, but still!). Then I would put my tray down and go for some soup and bread. When I sat at the table I had quite a spread in front of me. I got busy chatting and eating and before not too long my plate was empty. One by one my friends got up to for seconds. Often, I would join unaware of whether I was hungry or not. All that changed when I became mindful. Instead of just piling food on I checked in with myself as to how hungry I was and what I really wanted to eat. Then I would choose the foods I preferred in amounts that made sense to my level of hunger at that time.

Sometimes I knew I would want some protein with my lunch and since this buffet didn't offer protein, I would bring a can or two of salmon with me to toss in. My friends noticed what I was doing and became curious. I shared with them my decision to become a mindful eater and soon they, too, were questioning their choices and portions. We continued to meet each month and support each other's efforts to be mindful. If buffets are intimidating places for you, plan to visit one within the next few weeks for a mindful experiment.

Here's what you do: (1) go when you are moderately hungry; (2) look over the food options before putting anything on your plate; (3) assess your level of hunger; (4) fill your plate with a modest amount of the foods you most want to eat—if you want to start with dessert, start there; (5) observe how you react to the temptations; (6) take your plate to the table; (7) sit down and do a mini-meditation; (8) eat what you have served yourself mindfully; (9) give yourself permission to go back to the buffet lines for more of whatever you want, noting how it feels to allow yourself more; (10) mindfully eat as much of the food as you want, paying attention to when you start to become full; (11) stop eating when you are moderately full, being sure to leave some food on your plates; and (12) take a moment to reflect on the meal you just ate and acknowledge yourself for engaging in this experiment.

***Today:* Do a mini-meditation before three meals or snacks, eat three meals or snacks mindfully and meditate for twenty-five minutes.**

***Today's Journal Question:* Journal how eating at a buffet mindfully differs from how you ate at a buffet in the past.**

JUNE 3:

HEALTHY EATING VS. DISORDERED EATING HABITS

If you have chosen the path of mindful eating, I believe it is because you have tried other ways to get your eating and weight "under control" and have failed to do so. I also believe that you have embraced, at one time or another, "healthy eating" as the road to success. You may have abandoned diets way before you discovered this approach and decided "just to eat healthy" but sadly that didn't work for you either. A primary reason why "just eating healthy" didn't work for you is because you most likely didn't change anything about your eating except the food you chose. What do I mean? Managing your weight in a way that is sustainable for a lifetime is not about what you eat. It is about how you eat. I know plenty of people who swear to me that they eat a good diet (and I believe them) but they eat that "good diet" in a disordered way. Let me give you an example. The current version of the Weight Watchers Program uses a point system to help dieters manage how much food they eat in a day.

All foods are given a point value and each Weight Watcher member is assigned a daily point total to consume. As long as they don't eat more than that number of points, they will achieve weight loss. To help their members eat more fruit and vegetables, these foods are given no point values. They are "free." Here's where one of my clients went wrong. Because fruits have no points, she would eat a lot of fruit. Eating fruit is a good habit but not when you are eating it just to eat it. In other words, this client was not eating fruit in response to her body's need for fruit; she was eating fruit in response to her need to eat. She was eating fruit whenever she wanted to eat, period. Because they have no points, she thought she what she was doing was okay but when the scale failed to register any weight loss the error of her ways became apparent. Her fruit eating was "disordered eating." She was not in touch with her body's Inner Wisdom and was eating fruit regardless of whether she was hungry or full. I encouraged her to stay with the Weight Watchers program if she felt it was valuable to her but to use mindful eating habits as the foundation of her approach to food. Fruits might have zero points but even zero points is too many points if the body doesn't need them.

Today: **Do a mini-meditation before three meals or snacks, eat three meals or snacks mindfully and meditate for twenty-five minutes.**

Today's Journal Question: **What is the difference for you between healthy and disordered eating?**

JUNE 4:
FOODS THAT PULL

Along your journey to becoming a mindful eater you will become more aware of food. You will have a better understanding of which foods you enjoy, which foods your body prefers, which foods you can leave behind. There will be some food which dominate. Foods which call your name. Foods you must have, can't resist and can never get enough of. I call these foods "Foods that Pull." Don't feel bad if this far into your journey, you have "foods that pull." It's normal. We all have them. These foods are foods usually associated with something meaningful. They may represent a wonderful time in your life, a treasured memory, a cherished friend or relative or a source of great comfort.

A food that pulls me is mac and cheese. Mac and cheese is my go-to food when I need "that loving feeling." When I think about why mac and cheese, I think about my childhood. My parents are immigrants and when my mother came to the United States in the 1950s, packaged, processed foods were all the rage. She became an expert on making Rice-A-Roni, Shake and Bake, Stouffer's TV dinners and Kraft's Macaroni and Cheese. My favorite was the Kraft's. When she made it, I felt happy and loved. I formed an association between that food and feeling good so, later in life when I wanted that good feeling, I sought out mac and cheese. I came to understand this habit as I learned more about emotional eating, and I became really aware of it as I grew into mindful eating. Before I became a mindful eater, I gave myself permission to have mac and cheese when I wanted it, understanding that it was serving an important need. If you are familiar with my work around emotional eating you know that I never tell people not to eat. I would serve myself a portion of mac and cheese to feel better. And it worked. It wasn't until I became a mindful eater that I recognized that while it worked, it didn't taste good. When I really tasted the mac and cheese, it tasted like chemicals!

Now when I feel a pull towards mac and cheese, I make a different choice. Yes, I choose to have some if I really want it but I now choose a different version. I serve a homemade version which I prepare myself or buy from a specialty market; no more processed, nasty-tasting mac and cheese from a box. Now I offer myself only the best mac and cheese I can find and savor every bite of it in a mindful way.

If you have foods that pull, I want you to do two things. First, recognize the reason for the pull. Why that food? Why at that time? If you can address the underlying meaning of that food in another way than eating, give that way a try. If you want to have that food, have it, but do so mindfully.

Which brings me to the second thing I want you to do. Choose your favorite version of the food that pulls (if you love the box version, go for it) and eat your choice mindfully. You do not need to hide eating it. You do not need to eat it fast because you feel wrong for having it. Savor it as you would any other food. A mindfully eaten food that pulls is a way to offer yourself healing, kindness and support.

***Today:* Do a mini-meditation before three meals or snacks, eat three meals or snacks mindfully and meditate for twenty-five minutes.**

***Today's Journal Question:* What foods pull you?**

JUNE 5:
YOU ARE NOT A BAD PERSON

Becoming a Mindful Eater is a work in progress. It is an effortful journey that will have its easy times and its struggles. You do not become a Mindful Eater overnight. And you will never be a "perfect" mindful eater. Your goal is eating mindfully more often than not. Getting to that goal takes time, practice, patience, and self-compassion. By pursuing mindful eating, you are very likely giving up habits that have been a part of the fabric of your life for decades. Give yourself a break! If you are wrestling with any aspect of mindfulness or mindful eating, that's okay. We all do. The only way you can truly fail is to give up. If you go days, weeks, even months eating mindlessly, so what? Today, you can eat one bite mindfully. Today, you can sit for one minute in meditation. You are not a bad person if you are having a hard time. You are not a failure or someone who is doomed to always eat mindlessly. The fact that you still have this book in your hand is a testament to your efforts. Give yourself credit for what you have done. Have you tried to meditate? Good for you! Have you noticed when food tastes good and when it does not? Rock star! Have you eaten past fullness and been aware when you were doing so? That's being mindful! Pat yourself on your back for what you are trying to do and when you falter, pat yourself even more for noticing.

***Today:* Do a mini-meditation before three meals or snacks, eat three meals or snacks mindfully and meditate for twenty-five minutes.**

***Today's Journal Question:* In what way have you thought you were a bad person?**

JUNE 6:
WAITING FOR WEIGHT LOSS

I had lunch recently with a young colleague of mine. She's been a psychologist for about a year and a half and periodically we get together for a bit of mentoring. After talking about her work and advising her on the ins and outs of private practice, I told her about my new work with mindful eating. She was intrigued by the programs and coaching I am offering and then asked me the question everyone asks me when they hear about mindful eating, "What about weight loss?" I told her what I tell others. Mindful eating is a non-diet approach to weight management that is not a quick fix, but rather has the potential to be a permanent one.

Then I asked her the question I pose at the beginning of every mindful eating program, "How would you feel if a year from now you have lost some, not as much as you might have wanted but still some, and you know that the weight is off for good?"

Without hesitation, her eyes opened wide, and she said, "Tremendous! That would be great. Who wouldn't want that?"

Exactly. If you have been practicing your mindful eating skills and doing your daily meditations, and have not yet lost the weight you want to lose, please be patient. It is coming. I know it can be frustrating when all you want is the weight off, but haven't you lost weight before and it returned? Sometimes with a bonus pound or two? Release the goal of weight loss for the time being and concentrate on obtaining peace with food and peace of mind. The weight will come off. Remember, a watched pot never boils!

***Today:* Do a mini-meditation before three meals or snacks, eat three meals or snacks mindfully and meditate for twenty-five minutes.**

***Today's Journal Question:* What can you do to give yourself time to get the weight off?**

JUNE 7:
EVEN SEASONED MEDITATORS FALTER

To gain the benefits of meditation, you have to do it! Even meditators who have been practicing for years have to keep urging themselves to practice. I once had a teacher who said she fought getting onto her cushion each morning. She also told a story about a highly esteemed teacher of hers who "confessed" the same truth. I don't know about you, but her disclosure was comforting to me. It becomes hard to meditate regularly when we are faced with obstacles that get in our way, such as time and location. Other impediments can arise during the practice itself, making it less than pleasant or downright uncomfortable. These include: sleepiness, body aches, restlessness and unwanted emotions. Here are some tips to help your overcome these challenges.

If you feel sleepy, do your meditation with your eyes opened slightly. The light that enters your pupils will help you stay awake. If you are feeling physical discomfort, focus your attention on the source of your pain. It may seem counterintuitive, but resting your attention on your pain helps it go away. If you are restless, develop an attitude of curiosity towards your restlessness. Explore it. If you really can't sit still, shift to a walking meditation in which the focus of your attention is each step. Finally, if unwanted emotions come up during your meditation, try being present with them. Notice the thoughts and bodily sensations that accompany them. By focusing on them with lightness and wonder, they become easier to tolerate. If they are too intense or traumatic, seek psychotherapy to help resolve them. Whatever difficulties you face, keep practicing, because mixed in with the tough days will be glorious ones which I wouldn't want you to miss.

***Today:* Do a mini-meditation before three meals or snacks, eat three meals or snacks mindfully and meditate for twenty-five minutes.**

***Today's Journal Question:* How can knowing that even seasoned meditators struggle with their practice help you?**

JUNE 8:
IT'S WHAT YOU DO MOST OF THE TIME THAT COUNTS

Do you suffer from the "disease" of perfectionism? If you don't do everything right, do you think you do everything wrong? If you eat even one bite off your "food plan," do you toss in the towel? Believing that you need to be perfect is common. For some, the need starts in childhood, sprung from the notion that if you are perfect, you will be loved. For others it develops as a coping mechanism against poor self-esteem. Regardless of its origins, striving for perfection is a useless pursuit. You do not need to be perfect to experience success. Let's take baseball as an example. Baseball players are ranked using their batting averages. A batting average is the number of hits a batter has divided by the number of times he is at bat. The best baseball players in the world have batting averages around .350 (Ty Cobb's was .366 and Babe Ruth's was .342). This means that for every ten baseballs pitched at them, these batters hit the ball 3.5 times.

That means they missed 6.5 times. Hardly perfect and yet these are the best of the best. You don't need to hit the ball each time it's tossed, either, to be successful. It is what you do most of the time that makes the difference. If more often than not you are eating mindfully, you are doing great. If you meditate most days, awesome! Reflect on your habits and see what you do most. Are these habits that help you achieve your goals of health and weight loss or do they hinder you? If you stay up until 2 a.m. every night and get only four hours of sleep is that helping or hurting you? Practice mindful eating and mindfulness most of the time and you will be well on your way to successful weight loss and healthy habits.

Today: **Do a mini-meditation before three meals or snacks, eat three meals or snacks mindfully and meditate for twenty-five minutes.**

Today's Journal Question: **What do you do "most of the time" that serves you or hurts you?**

JUNE 9:

MY SISTER AND THE HOT DOG

During my transition to mindful eating, I went back east to visit my parents at the Senior Community where they were living. One of the days of my visit was Grandparents Day and the entire community celebrated with a barbecue. Before I got onto the lunch line, I snuck a peek at what was being offered. The choices were coleslaw, potato salad, corn the cob, hamburgers, hot dogs, watermelon, and ice cream bars. When it was my turn, I selected a little bit of the coleslaw, a little bit of the potato salad, a hamburger with a bun and a plain hot dog. I took a seat between my sister and my mother and prepared to eat my meal. I tasted a small portion of the coleslaw. It was okay, but not great. I did the same with the potato salad. It was tastier than the coleslaw. I took a bite of the hamburger and it was pretty good.

Then, I took a bite from the hot dog and yuck, awful. I turned to my sister and asked "Did you try the hot dog? It's nasty." Before she could answer I took another bite.

She saw me do that and remarked with a smile, "If it's so nasty, why did you take another bite? That's not being mindful."

I swallowed and with a soft chuckle in my voice answered, "I had to be sure!" As soon as I said that we both started laughing.

Between giggles, she asked, "Are you sure now?"

I said, "I sure am" and tossed the hot dog into the nearest trash bin.

I share this story with you so can learn from it. When you are at a barbecue or buffet, take a moment to review the selections offered and mindfully decide what your choices will be. It's okay to take some of each item if that's what you want. Be particular and selective. Choose what you want. If what you chose is not to your liking, replace it or toss it. You don't have to eat food that doesn't taste good to you. You may be thinking, "But what if all that was offered were those awful hot dogs?" If that were the case, I would have had two choices. First, I could have chosen to not eat and waited until later when I could have eaten something else. If that were not an option because I was physically hungry and I knew that it would be a long time before I could eat something else, I could have eaten the hot dog with full awareness that I am doing so because I am physically hungry, my body needs fuel and I want to feed it. It's okay to eat less than ideal foods or eat under less than ideal conditions. As long as you do so with your full awareness, you are being mindful.

***Today:* Do a mini-meditation before three meals or snacks, eat three meals or snacks mindfully and meditate for twenty-five minutes.**

***Today's Journal Question:* What could you do when you are faced with foods selections that are sub-par?**

JUNE 10:
MINDFUL EATING WITH FAMILY AND FRIENDS

June is a month typically filled with gatherings. From Father's Day to graduations and weddings, there are usually many occasions to be eating around friends and family. So, how do you eat mindfully in such situations? It depends. It depends upon whether or not you have already shared your mindful eating journey with them. It depends on how comfortable you are sharing what you are doing. And it depends upon how open they may be to learn what you are learning. If your family and friends know about your great mindful eating adventure, then keep doing what you are doing. Eat when you are hungry, stop when you are full and choose the foods that are right for you. If you have not shared the changes you are working on, now might be a nice time to do so. You can explain that you have embarked on a new approach to food and eating and that you have been building mindful eating skills for the past several months.

You can explain to them that mindful eating means eating with full attention, savoring your food and honoring your body. You can tell them about the changes that are happening and how much more peaceful you feel around food. On the other hand, if you are not comfortable sharing what you are doing, then don't. There is no need to draw attention to your new habits if you don't want to or feel as if they will not be received well. In those cases, just quietly go about your mindful eating business. If people notice that you are not eating or are leaving food on your plate and they question you, you can simply say that you've had enough, it doesn't taste so good or you are not hungry. If people insist on pushing food on you, ask if you can take it home so you can it enjoy later. Then when you are home you can decide whether it is food you want to keep or toss. Whatever approach you take, I encourage you to savor not only the food but also the time with family and friends. Be mindful of the love that surrounds and the joy that each occasion brings.

***Today:* Do a mini-meditation before three meals or snacks, eat three meals or snacks mindfully and meditate for twenty-five minutes.**

***Today's Journal Question:* How might you introduce your mindful eating journey to your family and friends?**

JUNE 11:

MAKING CHOICES THAT LEAD TO WHERE YOU WANT TO GO

It is often said that the shortest distance between two points is a straight line. If only that were true about life. I don't know about you, but rarely has my life followed a straight line—well, maybe until high school and then the zigzagging began. I didn't have a straight line into psychology. You may recall I had an entire career in law first. My weight didn't fall into place with the first diet I ever tried. It took years and many missteps to get to mindful eating. What kept me going and eventually reaching where I wanted to go was keeping my eye on the prize. I knew I wanted a career where I thrived, one that matched my personality and allowed me to help people in a significant way. For me, law did not fit the bill so I investigated other choices and decided on psychology. Best decision I ever made. True, I got to this career ten years later than I wish I had, but I got here and have been happy ever since. Same thing with my weight. I went on my first diet at fifteen. Looking back, I can see that I wasn't heavy, but teenage girls diet and so did I. Little did I know then that dieting causes weight gain. Who knows what might have happened had I never stepped onto that merry-go-round? But I did and I gained weight and lost weight and gained again. I was at my heaviest in law school where I ate peanut M&M's as a coping mechanism.

Not knowing about emotional eating and how to properly address it, I continued to diet. (I write about this in *The Best Diet Begins in Your Mind*). Once I learned about healing emotional eating and taking a non-diet approach to weight management, my weight went down again until I started perimenopause. I suffered for seventeen years with symptoms (and thirty excess pounds) before I graduated into menopause. It was during this episode of my life that I found mindful eating and restored my body back to its right size. Straight line? Nope. Focused effort? Definitely. Each day to the best of my ability I make choices that lead me to where I want to go. With regards to my eating, that means I make mindful choices that lead me to peace with food and the right weight for me. Even without a straight line you can get to where you want to go by keeping your eye on the prize and taking the kind of action that can get you there.

***Today:* Do a mini-meditation before three meals or snacks, eat three meals or snacks mindfully and meditate for twenty-five minutes.**

***Today's Journal Question:* What can you do to help yourself stay focused and make the kind of choices that lead to peace with food and the right weight for you?**

JUNE 12:
DOWN AND OUT

I hope that by now you have come to discover that being a mindful eater is about so much more than losing weight. I hope that by now you are experiencing a level of comfortableness around food that you may never have felt before, are coping with your emotions without always using food, and are naturally eating less. If weight loss is still your number one goal, and you are feeling a bit impatient, then it is time to consider where else you could cut down or cut out some of the food you are currently eating. For example, perhaps you are still ending the day with a dish of ice cream, and may be now you are eating it in a pretty bowl at your table after doing a mini-meditation. That's all good. But maybe you don't need to eat the ice cream every night. Maybe that serving of ice cream is a form of emotional eating. If that's the case, find another way to unwind, perhaps a bath, a book or a foot rub. If you do want the ice cream, how about choosing a brand that you enjoy but has less fat or maybe serving it in a cup rather than a bowl so you naturally take a smaller portion? Think about where you might make some cuts without feeling deprived and when you are ready, make such a cut and see what happens.

Today: **Do a mini-meditation before three meals or snacks, eat three meals or snacks mindfully and meditate for twenty-five minutes.**

Today's Journal Question: **If you are feeling impatient about your weight loss, why is that?**

JUNE 13:

RELAX YOUR BODY AND YOUR MIND WILL FOLLOW

In one of the mindfulness classes I attended, I was taught how important it is to learn to relax. While mindfulness meditation is not specifically a tool for relaxation, learning to calm the body helps to calm the mind. As the teacher Elisha Goldstein, PhD, said, "When we strengthen the skill of relaxing the body, the mind tends to follow." As our mind and body unwind, we are better able to be present to what is around us and to focus and concentrate on what needs our attention. Can you see how this might support your mindful eating? Not only are you less likely to stress eat, you are also more likely to manage all of your emotions in a healthier way. Find a way to relax your body on a daily basis. You might simply lie down and take five deep breaths through your nose and out through your mouth and as you do, imagine all the stress in your body dissolving. See it flowing out of your fingertips and toes or evaporating from the crown of your head.

Today: **Do a mini-meditation before three meals or snacks, eat three meals or snacks mindfully and meditate for twenty-five minutes.**

Today's Journal Question: **How can learning to relax help you?**

JUNE 14:

OUTER GUIDANCE—CLEAN EATING

There are many forms of Outer Guidance that may assist you in becoming a mindful eater, losing weight and achieving good health. One option is to consider "clean eating." Author of *The Eat-Clean Diet* Tosca Reno defines clean eating as avoiding processed, prepackaged and fast foods and building a diet around fresh fruits and vegetables, whole grains, lean proteins and heathy fats. The simplest way to implement clean eating is to eliminate processed foods from your diet. What are processed foods? My definition—anything with words on the label you can't produce or neither heard of. You don't have to switch to a clean diet overnight. That's not necessarily being mindful. Instead try a clean meal or snack and see how you feel. Is clean eating a good choice for you? If it is, how can you incorporate more clean food into your diet? If you like to cook you can find recipes online. If you don't like to cook, many health food stores (like Whole Foods) offer prepared clean foods. If clean eating isn't for you, no worries. Remember with mindful eating, you get to choose.

Today: **Do a mini-meditation before three meals or snacks, eat three meals or snacks mindfully and meditate for twenty-five minutes.**

Today's Journal Question: **Is clean eating a form of Outer Guidance that you might like to experiment with, and why or why not?**

JUNE 15:

GIRLS JUST WANNA HAVE FUN

In 1983 mega-star Cyndi Lauper released the hit song, "Girls Just Wanna Have Fun." If you are old enough to remember that song, I am sure you are humming it right now. (I am singing it in my head as I write these words for you.) If you were not around in 1983, listen to it on iTunes. Great song. Lots of fun. I bring up Cyndi's sang because I want to make sure you are having some fun in your life. We are a world of busy bees. Our days are so filled up with work, family obligations and community service we often leave very little time for ourselves. It is important to make time for play, for fun. A mindful life is a full life and a full life includes joy, laughter and silliness. Make time for play. See a movie. Tease your cat with a flashlight. Watch a comedy. Ride bikes with your kids. Have date night with your partner. When we play, we learn to take things lightly, to be present in the moment and feel joy. If we take ourselves and our lives too seriously, we fall prey to mindlessness, robotically churning out chore after chore, duty after duty. Play allows us to pause and be in the moment. Play makes room for mindfulness. Play today.

***Today:* Do a mini-meditation before three meals or snacks, eat three meals or snacks mindfully and meditate for twenty-five minutes.**

***Today's Journal Question:* How can you play today?**

JUNE 16:
COURAGE TO CHANGE

We are all afraid of something. I have a fear of heights. I am fine in an airplane or elevator but I could never peer over a cliff or stand on the ledge of anything. Not all fears are about physical conditions like that. Some fears are about circumstances, like public speaking. Some are about emotions, like anger or grief. And sometimes the thing we fear is change. The fear of change can be especially debilitating, because as French nobleman and author Francois de la Rochefoucauld said, "The only thing constant in life is change." Everything changes. Green leaves turn brown in autumn. Puppies become dogs. Children grow up. Hair goes gray. When you are the object of change, people around you may feel uncomfortable.

They want you to stay the same. You may want to stay the same because it feels, in the moment, easier. But change is inevitable and when you learn to accept it life becomes fuller. I welcome change because I know that it will arrive invited or not. I know that with change comes new experiences, new opportunities for growth, even if that change is painful—such as death or illness. We face fear and change with courage. Changing your eating habits to mindful ones takes courage. You are flying in the face of societal norm to eat mindlessly and emotionally. But you can do it. Making changes such as these builds confidence. When you know that you can eat mindfully in all situations, you are empowered to take on other challenges. I encourage you to not be afraid of change, but to embrace it. Befriend it rather than fear it because as hard as you try, you cannot avoid it

***Today:* Do a mini-meditation before three meals or snacks, eat three meals or snacks mindfully and meditate for twenty-five minutes.**

***Today's Journal Question:* How might the fear of change hold you back?**

JUNE 17:
ARE YOU EATING FOR YOUR BEST EVERY-THING?

A lovely side effect of using mindful eating as your tool for weight loss is that it has the potential to positively affect your entire life. Your sense of self, purpose and attitude towards your body can improve. But there is one caveat—you need to consistently listen to and honor your Inner Wisdom. As you have learned, your Inner Wisdom is that wise part of yourself that knows what is best for you. When you tune into it, it will lead you to the right food, the right amounts, the right timing and the right movement for your body's needs. Each time you make such a mindful choice you are eating for your best everything.

The integrity that follows the mindful eating path is life-changing. You learn that you can depend upon yourself to do what is in your best interest and you demonstrate to yourself and others that you are a person of your word. As you cultivate mindfulness in all its facets, your life shifts from one ruled by reaction, chaos, confusion and pain to one guided by calm, purpose, intention and peace. So, from now on, each time you take a mindful bite or sit for meditation, you can have confidence in that moment that you are doing what is best for you, all of you.

***Today:* Do a mini-meditation before three meals or snacks, eat three meals or snacks mindfully and meditate for twenty-five minutes.**

***Today's Journal Question:* How will you take an action today that is for your best everything?**

JUNE 18:
CELEBRATE YOUR MISTAKES

I have a secret for you—no one is perfect. No one becomes a mindful eater overnight, and certainly no one never eats mindlessly. At least no human I have ever met and that includes me. "Mistakes" happen. In the past when you made a "mistake" on your diet (usually referred to as "cheating"), that may have meant the end of your efforts. If not the end permanently, then it most likely led to an interim period of condemnation, self-criticism and judgment before resuming the diet. Not anymore. There are no "mistakes" in mindful eating. You are either mindful or you are not, and if you are not that is not a mistake. A moment when you are not being mindful is a moment for observation, curiosity and self-reflection. When you notice that you are not being mindful, celebrate because in that moment of noticing you are, in fact, being mindful! It is a moment of victory, not failure. Mindfulness is all about living in the here and now. Of observing, without judgment, what is happening and learning from it. So, the next time you make a "mistake" whatever that mistake may be, celebrate it for the gift it is—a moment of mindfulness from which you can gain clarity and make another choice.

***Today:* Do a mini-meditation before three meals or snacks, eat three meals or snacks mindfully and meditate for twenty-five minutes.**

***Today's Journal Question:* How have you reacted to "mistakes" in the past and what might you do differently now?**

JUNE 19:
MEDITATION MAKE US MORE RESILIENT

Have you ever noticed that when you are in a good mood life seems easier? Events that might otherwise irritate you, say traffic or a slow elevator, barely register. On the other hand, when you are in a bad mood, nothing goes right. Most situations are annoying or aggravating. Even the little things, like not having a postage stamp when you need one, become monumental. The skill necessary to bounce back from difficulties is called resiliency. A willow tree is a beautiful example. When caught in a storm, the willow tree bends all the way to the ground yielding to the power of the wind and sways upright when the wind passes. We can do that too. We can learn to move with the storms in our lives and remain intact and whole.

Our tool for building resiliency is mindfulness meditation, of course. Our minds have what researchers call a negative bias. We are prone to see and react to the negative. Our brains light up with more neural activity when negative events are presented than when positive ones appear. From an evolutionary perspective this is vital. We need to be alert and ready to respond to threats. However, in today's world what many of us might perceive as threats are not the kind of threats our biology is expecting. A traffic jam is different than a saber-toothed tiger. Fortunately, we don't live in a world filled with such dangers, but we do have our own versions—stock market crashes, cancer, divorce. Building the skill of resiliency through meditation can serve you well when faced with our 21st century opponents. In your meditation practice continue to watch your thoughts without hanging on to them. Let them float by like clouds in a breezy sky. Not attaching to negative thoughts helps keep you in a positive frame of mind, which as we know makes life easier to tolerate.

***Today:* Do a mini-meditation before three meals or snacks, eat three meals or snacks mindfully and meditate for twenty-five minutes.**

***Today's Journal Question:* How resilient are you?**

JUNE 20:

ARE YOU ADDICTED TO STIMULATION?

There is an invisible epidemic sweeping our world. Do you know what it is? It's a world-wide addiction to stimulation. Since cell phones and technology devices have become commonplace, people are getting used to being constantly engaged in something. Whether it is texting, talking, emailing, listing to music, watching videos, or playing games, people are seeking constant stimulation. Without something grabbing their attention they feel lost, out of sorts, uneasy, even anxious. And it's not just teens. I know plenty of adults who can't get off Facebook or won't stop playing Candy Crush if their life depended on it, and in many ways, it does.

The problem with this constant need for stimulation is that it makes it hard for people to be still. When clients complain to me that they can't meditate, this is often a primary reason. Being attached to our favorite gadget leaves us isolated from human contact and for some a loss of meaning or purpose in life. Where would your mind be if you weren't distracted by your source of stimulation? What would you be thinking? What would you be doing? Creating? Building? And with whom would you be doing it? Take a chance and put down your phone. Sit quietly and allow your mind to wander to all the beautiful places, people and opportunities the world has to offer. Seek a life of greater meaning and deeper connections than what a text message can give you. When you do, I suspect you will eat less and enjoy life more.

***Today:* Do a mini-meditation before three meals or snacks, eat three meals or snacks mindfully and meditate for twenty-five minutes.**

***Today's Journal Question:* If you are addicted to stimulation, how has it affected your life and your weight?**

JUNE 21:
MINDLESS MOMENTS

Recently I had a series of mindless moments that made me stop, pause, and breathe. Let me explain. I spent most of the day at home writing. To take a break I decided to run to the supermarket for a few items. I grabbed two reusable grocery bags and my keys and I drove off. I parked my car and as I opened the car door to get out, I reached for my purse. It was in that moment I realized I had left the house without my purse. That meant I left the house without my wallet, which meant, among other things, I was driving without a license. Yeesh! I rolled my eyes, smiled at myself in the rearview mirror, pulled the car door shut and drove home. Mindless moment #1.

When I got home, I ran up the stairs, yanked the purse off the counter, got back into the car and returned to the store. A few minutes later, as I was blissfully walking among the store aisles to retrieve the items I needed, I noticed for the first time I had left my shopping list on the fridge door. Another eye roll, followed by a sigh and deep breath. Mindless moment #2. I continued with my shopping as best I could, trying to remember what was written on my list. When I had what I thought I needed, I proceeded to the cashier. I placed a reusable bag and my items on the counter and placed the basket I had been carrying atop a pile of other baskets. After swiping my credit card, I took my bag and went home. I unloaded the groceries placing each item in its rightful place and folded up the grocery bag. It was then that I realized I had left the second reusable bag in the basket at the store. Mindless moment #3. I shook my head in disbelief. Three mindless moments within the span of an hour. What was going on? Instead of berating myself, I got curious. Why was I so forgetful this afternoon? I rarely, if ever, leave the house without my purse or shopping list or leave anything in a store. I took a few deep calming breaths and reflected on my day. I recognized that I was preoccupied. Even though my body was shopping, my mind was somewhere else, specifically on the pages of this book.

Now, don't get me wrong, dear reader, I am not blaming you. I am saying that my mind was so focused on my writing I was not present for my shopping. Has that ever happened to you? You are so focused on one task that you "forget" something else. If it has, you had a mindless moment. Mindless moments happen. The important thing is to not beat yourself up but rather to be curious and compassionate about what happened. Mindless moments happened when we are rushing, preoccupied, trying to do too many things at once. To prevent mindless moments, slow down, take your time and be mindful.

Today: **Do a mini-meditation before three meals or snacks, eat three meals or snacks mindfully and meditate for twenty-five minutes.**

Today's Journal Question: **What mindless moments did you have today?**

JUNE 22:
CHANGE YOUR STORY, CHANGE YOUR LIFE

We are what we think about most. We are the stories we tell about ourselves. What stories do you tell about yourself? Do you tell yourself you are an emotional eater? You will always be fat? The story you tell yourself makes up your self-image. If your self-image is that you fail at weight loss and are destined to be overweight like the rest of your family, you will have a hard time getting the weight of and keeping it off. Let me give you an example from a different point of view. Lottery winners. Did you know that most of lottery winners will lose their winnings? It's true. I have seen statistics that say at least 70% of lottery winners are broke within seven years. You may ask yourself, why does that happen? The answer, from a psychological perspective, is that these winners did not see themselves as wealthy people. In their heart of hearts, they were still poor. This creates a state of mind known as cognitive dissonance.

Cognitive dissonance happens when a person holds two contrary beliefs. In the case of the lottery winners, the conflicting thoughts are, "I am rich and I am poor." For the person trying to change her weight, the conflict may be, "I am fat and I am thin." If you want to succeed on this journey, we are taking, I want to encourage you to change your story. Change your narrative. Change how you see yourself. Start thinking about yourself as a mindful eater, a meditator, and a person who has healthy coping skills. Gather evidence of your new self-image. Review your meditation log for proof you are a meditator. Look at your journal for confirmation that you are becoming a mindful eater. Work with your self-image as you practice the skills you are learning. A shift in your self-image will go a long way to shift your weight.

Today: **Do a mini-meditation before three meals or snacks, eat three meals or snacks mindfully and meditate for twenty-five minutes.**

Today's Journal Question: **Write a new description of your self-image which reflects your goal of losing weight through mindful eating.**

JUNE 23:
EASY DOES IT

If you have been following this journey day by day, today is day 174. Congratulations! Well done! Over these past 174 days you may have wondered why I designed this journey to be 365 days. True, I could have given you all this information upfront for you to digest over a few days or weeks, but that wouldn't have given you the time you really need to make mindful eating and mindfulness second nature. Change takes time. Nothing, no amount of instruction, encouragement or guidance, takes the place of time. Time gives you a chance to ease into this transformation. Time gives you room to practice, learn and apply what works for you and what doesn't.

Time opens up space for the inevitable obstacles to arise. By going slowly and creating a sense of ease around this process, you become better equipped to handle a setback without giving up. You know from experience how to acknowledge with curiosity what is occurring and to gently bring yourself back to the present. Time also gives you room to adapt mindfulness into your lifestyle in a way that suits you best. That's why this is a one-year journey. If you are feeling rushed or impatient with this process, stop, breathe. Ask yourself, why the rush? Why the urgency? Approach your answers with mindful attention and observe what happens. There is a famous quote attributed to Maya Angelou: "All great achievements require time." Becoming a mindful eater is a great achievement. Give yourself the gift of time.

***Today:* Do a mini-meditation before three meals or snacks, eat three meals or snacks mindfully and meditate for twenty-five minutes.**

***Today's Journal Question:* How might going slowly and taking this transformation into becoming a mindful eater slowly help you achieve your goals?**

JUNE 24:
LET IT BE

I was about three years old when The Beatles first appeared on the Ed Sullivan Show. I didn't see them then because I wasn't old enough, but in the decades that followed I did see that appearance and many more. I became a big fan. Among my favorite Beatle songs is Let it Be. That song is about a vision of the Virgin Mary (referred to as Mother Mary) offering wisdom to the singer by encouraging him to let the troubles that plague him be. Those lyrics echo three messages inherent in a mindfulness practice – wisdom, acceptance, and non-attachment. In the song, Mother Mary represents guiding wisdom. In our mindfulness work, we use our Inner Wisdom to guide us. And the words "let it be" reflect the mindfulness principles of acceptance and non-attachment to outcome. When you find yourself in trouble because you are eating too much, running late for work, or have a hole in your sock, remember the words "let it be" and allow your Inner Wisdom and meditation practice to guide you.

***Today:* Do a mini-meditation before three meals or snacks, eat three meals or snacks mindfully and meditate for twenty-five minutes.**

***Today's Journal Question:* Find a recording of Let it Be and reflect on how letting things be can serve your mindful eating process.**

JUNE 25:
THINK LIKE A GENIUS

Albert Einstein is credited with saying, "You never fail until you stop trying." I couldn't agree more. In some ways I live by that motto. When asked once what I would want written on my tombstone, I quipped, "She tried!" On my journey to a healthy relationship with food, I tried a lot of different methods. I tried dieting the old-fashioned way. I tried studying the research on food addiction. I tried various treatment protocols for ending emotional eating. I experimented on myself until I found what works for me—mindful eating. If I hadn't kept trying, if I had given up after the first diet, you wouldn't be reading this and I wouldn't have found my life's work. When in your life have you failed because you stopped trying? What have you accomplished because you didn't stop trying? A college degree? A happy marriage? Children? The perfect parking space? Put the same tenacity you put into achieving something that felt unattainable to your mindful eating efforts and see what happens. As long as you are trying, you are not failing.

***Today:* Do a mini-meditation before three meals or snacks, eat three meals or snacks mindfully and meditate for twenty-five minutes.**

***Today's Journal Question:* How can you tap into your genius today?**

JUNE 26:

WEIGHTY LESSONS

When someone comes to me for psychotherapy about his or her weight problem, I would explain that my approach to this issue is to look for the answer to this question: Why does this person overeat? Some eat to stay overweight because they need the weight for some reason. Others overeat for emotional reasons and the consequence is the excess weight but the real problem is not the weight, the real problem is the emotional eating. For a few, both answers are true. So far, we have been looking at emotional eating; today I want to look at what purpose being overweight may be serving for you. On the surface it might seem obvious that being in a "right-sized" body would be preferable to being in an "over-sized" body, but as you well know, things are not always as they appear. For some people carrying excess weight is preferable because that excess weight serves some purpose for them.

Figuring out what that purpose is and what to do about it is helpful. Among the reasons I have heard are: being larger make people notice them, being heavy makes them invisible, and extra weight keeps them safe. Interesting, each of these reasons can be addressed without needing a bigger sized body. Small people get noticed or stay invisible. A person can learn to be safe by becoming more assertive or learning martial arts. In addition, excess weight can teach us. It can teach us that we don't have good coping skills, or that we need more Outer Guidance on healthy foods choices, or that we watch too much TV. When you figure out what purpose your excess weight is serving, or what lesson it is trying to teach, you can use your mindfulness-based skills and tools to address it. One caveat—please keep in mind that this mindful journey is not psychotherapy. If you feel psychotherapy would be appropriate for you, go to the Psychology Today website to find a psychologist near you. Look for someone who specializes in eating issues, preferably someone with a mindful eating slant.

Today: **Do a mini-meditation before three meals or snacks, eat three meals or snacks mindfully and meditate for twenty-five minutes.**

Today's Journal Question: **What did/does your weight teach you?**

JUNE 27:

DIFFERENT KINDS OF BREATH

We all know how to breathe but did you know that there are different ways to breathe? There is the Whisper Breath which is a slow "ha" sound, as if you were fogging up a mirror. There is Breath of Fire breathing with forced inhales and exhales. There is Chant Breathing which repeats the word "Om" as you exhale. There is Alternative Nostril Breathing during which you alternate breathing through your nostril by pinching closed the one you are not using. Each type of breath creates a different physiological response in your body that can be used for healing. Breathing has been shown to improve sleep, decrease the stress hormone cortisol and alleviate depression. Practice each of them to see how they make you feel.

***Today:* Do a mini-meditation before three meals or snacks, eat three meals or snacks mindfully and meditate for twenty-five minutes.**

***Today's Journal Question:* How can you use breathing to restore your well-being?**

JUNE 28:
LEARN THE ART OF STOPPING

In the book *Mindful Eating, Mindful Life* by Thich Nhat Hanh and Dr. Lilian Cheung, the authors talk about "the art of stopping." I love that phrase. If you think about it most of us are in forward motion all the time. We rush. We run. We flit from one task to another, from one conversation to another. We eat. The truth is we need to stop. We need to pause, take a breath and be present. When we stop, we can focus. When we focus, we can see. When we can see, we can heal. Stopping helps us live our best lives. Do you have trouble stopping? Is it hard for you to pause and take a moment to be still? Many people struggle with stopping because stillness frightens them. In the stillness thoughts and feelings emerge. Dark corners of their psyche reveal themselves and so they run. They get back into motion with such force that all unpleasantness is left in their dust. Sadly, other things are left in the dust too. Love, joy, passion and a full, satisfying life are often bypassed in the fury to stay busy. Keeping busy is just another form of mindlessness and as you already know mindlessness robs us of the present moment. Practice stopping today, if only for a minute, and see what happens.

***Today:* Do a mini-meditation before three meals or snacks, eat three meals or snacks mindfully and meditate for twenty-five minutes.**

Today's Journal Question: **If you typically rush through your day, what would happen if you stopped?**

JUNE 29:

ASSESS, ADJUST, ADVANCE

Tomorrow marks the end of six months on this journey of mindful eating. What is changing for you? How is your relationship to food and eating different than it was on January 1st? Assess the ways you are eating in a healthier, more mindful way. Adjust what you believe needs adjusting—an increased meditation practice, a better cushion, a new placemat to remind you to eat at a table. Reflect on these matters with an attitude of mindfulness, self-acceptance, and self-forgiveness for "not being perfect." Consider what you can do to advance in your journey. Then with gratitude for yourself and the effort you have be making, forge ahead.

Today: **Do a mini-meditation before three meals or snacks, eat three meals or snacks mindfully and meditate for twenty-five minutes.**

Today's Journal Question: **Write a paragraph or two about how your relationship to food has changed since January 1, acknowledging yourself as the source of these changes.**

JUNE 30:

I AM A FELLOW STRUGGLER

In case you are under the impression that mindful eating and mindful meditation come easy to me, I want to disavow you of that assumption. I too struggle. Not as much as when I first started, but still. I want you to know that it took me over a year and a half to establish a daily meditation practice. During those first eighteen months, I would start and stop on pretty much a daily basis. My best periods were when I was enrolled in a meditation class. Then I would keep up with the class assignments and practice daily but as soon as the class ended so would my daily practice until I began again. I embraced the principle of "begin again" like a precious heirloom. And it worked. Eventually I came to a daily practice. Well, I use the term daily loosely. Let's say an almost daily practice. A "most days" practice. And I am happy with that.

Ultimately, I would like to get to a twice a day practice. I trust that if I keep doing what I am doing that will come in time. As for my mindful eating, I am less than perfect. Like my meditation practice, my mindful eating habits developed in fits and starts. Because I kept at it, I can confidently call myself a mindful eater but it wasn't always easy. There were times when I was mindful. There were times when I was mindless and times when I was mindfully mindless (meaning I knew what I was doing was not mindful eating and I allowed myself to eat anyway.) No one is perfect nor should anyone aspire to that state. It can't be reached. We are all human and we have human frailties and imperfections. Embrace who you are and your process. Acknowledge yourself for your efforts whatever they are and keep on keeping on. You'll get there. Wherever there is.

Today: **Do a mini-meditation before three meals or snacks, eat three meals or snacks mindfully and meditate for twenty-five minutes.**

Today's Journal Question: **How can you acknowledge yourself for your efforts even if you are not doing as well as you might like to be?**

JULY

JULY 1:

EAT ALL YOUR MEALS AND SNACKS MINDFULLY

Today you will begin eating all your meals and snacks mindfully. What does that mean? This means:

1. As you prepare to eat your meal or snack, take a moment and get centered. Breathe. Focus your attention on this meal or snack. Do a mini-meditation if you like.
2. Check in with your hunger and make a mental note of where you are on your hunger scale.
3. Observe the food you have chosen to eat. Notice what it looks like, feels like, and smells like.
4. Think about the farmers, manufacturers, transportation vehicles, stock clerks, cashiers, and cooks who got this food to you. Silently thank them for their participation.
5. Eat your food slowly, paying attention to how it tastes and feels in your mouth.
6. Notice when/if the taste changes.
7. Check in with your fullness scale.
8. When you are comfortably full and satisfied, end your meal or snack and give yourself credit the mindful efforts you made.

At first this will feel cumbersome, but in time this approach will become second-natured and natural. Just like driving a car. When you first learned, you were hyperaware of every aspect. But now, you drive effortlessly. Mindful eating will be effortless too.

***Today:* Eat all your meals and snacks mindfully and meditate for twenty-five minutes.**

***Today's Journal Question:* How do you feel now that you are eating all your meals and snacks mindfully, or most of them anyway?**

JULY 2:
EXERCISE DOESN'T WORK FOR WEIGHT LOSS

What?! It's true. But what about all those mantras about calories in and calories out? Research is debunking those. Recent studies show us that exercise does not lead to weight loss the way we thought it did. Exercise is important for health but it is no longer touted as the panacea for weight loss. I introduced walking as a tool of mindfulness back in March but nowhere did I mention using walking for weight loss. Instead, I talked about stress reduction and mood enhancing. There is no question that exercise leads to better health—both physical and psychological. But for weight loss it is proving to be counterproductive.

One reason cited for why exercise for weight loss doesn't work is that when you exercise you end up eating more. Some exercisers are hungrier as a result of exercise and eat more, which would be okay if they were mindful about their hunger and fullness, but let's face it—most people are not. Eating more after exercise can lead to an increase in mindless eating which is contrary to our efforts. Another reason offered for why exercise is not a good method for weight loss is that it takes a lot of exercise to burn off enough calories to take the pounds off. For example, you would have to walk thirty-five miles to burn off 3,500 calories (the approximate amount you would need to lose pound). That's a lot of walking. Sure, you can do it. But in this journey, we are seeking balance. Trying to walk thirty-five miles a week to lose a pound seems unbalanced to me. All of this is not to say, don't exercise. It is to say don't exercise for weight loss. Mindfully separate the link between exercise and weight loss in your mind. Exercise because it feels good, addresses health concerns, improves sleep and improves your mood, not because you think it will quicken your weight loss efforts.

Today: **Eat all your meals and snacks mindfully and meditate for twenty-five minutes.**

Today's Journal Question: **What role has exercise played in your life?**

JULY 3:
GOOD TO THE LAST DROP

One day on my journey I noticed that I had a funny habit. Well, funny to me anyway. I noticed that when I was eating alone as soon as I took the last bite of whatever I was eating I would get up from the table and start putting the dishes away while still chewing. Up until that moment I was practicing mindful eating, noticing what I food I had chosen, how it tasted and so on. But as soon as that last bite went into my mouth, I went mindless. Funny, right? On that fateful day when I noticed I was doing this I became curious. Why did I do that? Why did I get up still chewing? Why did I go mindless at the last possible moment? As I pondered these questions it dawned on me that I was still having a hard time setting aside time to eat mindfully. As a habitual multi-tasker, stopping just to eat continued to be a challenge. I could do it for only so long until I felt the urge to jump up and get "back at it," whatever "it" was.

In the days that followed this revelation, I paid attention to when the urge to get "back at it" struck and when it didn't. A pattern emerged. On those days when I felt more rushed, pressed for time or eager to do something, I ate quicker and took that last bite mindlessly. On those days when I was more relaxed, at ease or had a more open schedule, I lingered over my food more and stayed at the table after the last bite. It occurred to me that this pattern happened when I did other things too. I would make mistakes if I rushed. I'd make typos, forget to buy an item at the store, get a papercut, ding my car, or leave something at home. In other words, rushing made me mindless. I made a decision to mindfully choose to slow down. To give myself more time to eat or to not eat if I didn't have the time to pay attention. To deliberately take my time doing tasks. To be more present at all times. Am I perfect at this? Nope. Am I getting better? Yep. Is it making a difference? It sure is. I am making fewer mistakes; no recent dings or papercuts and I am enjoying my food down to the very last drop.

***Today:* Eat all your meals and snacks mindfully and meditate for twenty-five minutes.**

***Today's Journal Question:* What are you still doing mindlessly that is affecting your eating, your body, and your life?**

JULY 4:

DECLARE YOUR INDEPENDENCE FROM FOOD WOES

If you are reading this in the United States, today is an important day. More than two hundred years ago, the United States of American declared its independence from England and established itself as a sovereign state. We typically celebrate this liberation with BBQs and fireworks. Today is great day for you to declare your own independence from whatever food and eating issues still plague you. Like our forefathers and foremothers, write a document declaring your freedom. In your journal, on your laptop or tablet, make a statement of what you would like to be free from. If you need some help doing this, here's a place to start.

I, ________________, declare myself to be free from mindless eating. I declare that I adopt a mindful approach to food and tap into the wisdom of my body and the knowledge of nutritional science to inform my food choices. I declare myself free from my previous eating habits which got in the way of my being my best self. I declare that I am a daily meditator and mindful eater. I declare that I savor my food and express appreciation for all those who contributed to its preparation. I declare myself free from emotional and stress eating and rely on more productive ways to manage my feelings. Finally, I declare that I offer myself and those around me compassion and gratitude on a regular basis. Signed this day, ___________________.

Don't worry if your freedom does not come overnight. Neither did America's. And like America, you are a work in progress.

***Today:* Eat all your meals and snacks mindfully and meditate for twenty-five minutes.**

***Today's Journal Question:* What will you declare your independence from today?**

JULY 5:

KEEP ON KEEPING ON

Twice before I have urged you to "keep on keeping on." Today makes three. I want to encourage you to continue being aware of the difference between physical and emotional hunger. Continue to evaluate your sensations of fullness and satisfaction. Continue savoring your food and tasting each bite. Continue to recognize your emotional or other triggers to lead you to eat or continue to eat. Wherever you are with these skills and habits is fine. Just remain steadfast on this journey. Doing what you can when you can and keep on keeping on.

***Today:* Eat all your meals and snacks mindfully and meditate for twenty-five minutes.**

***Today's Journal Question:* What mindful eating skills will you keep prac-**

ticing?

JULY 6:
GOAL SETTING

Thirty-five years or so ago I was in a place in my life when I was feeling lost and unsettled. I had just left my marriage, was in the middle of graduate school and finding it hard to get motivated about life. I reached out to a friend whom I knew was also suffering albeit for different reasons. I suggested we get together for lunch and set some goals for our lives. At lunch we set goals in each of following categories: Physical, Professional, Personal and Financial. Our goals were really modest—drink more water, study for finals (that was mine, hers were to see more clients), take a walk, cut coupons, etc. We agreed to meet a month later at the same restaurant to go over our goals. When we met the following month, we were both surprised that we had in fact done our respective goals. We set more goals and agreed to meet again in another month. We met again and once again had met our goals. This was working. We told two other friends what we were doing. They asked to join us and thus was born GSI—Goal Setting International. We called ourselves that because we set a goal of one day having our monthly meetings around the world!

We met regularly for years and reached all our goals—new jobs, new marriages, children, new careers, better health, and more wealth. I still attend GSI meetings although the membership has changed because among the goals of the original members was to move from Los Angeles, which they did! I am sharing GSI with you because I want to encourage you to set goals for yourself beyond mindful eating. Life is about more than food, diet and weight and I want you to have a great life. I believe that so strongly that I wrote an eBook called *Stop Dieting, Start Living* which shows you exactly how to do that. Consider setting some goals for yourself using the categories above. Maybe invite a friend or two to join you and establish your own GSI group. Make your life about more than your weight. You deserve it.

Today: **Eat all your meals and snacks mindfully and meditate for twenty-five minutes.**

Today's Journal Question: **What goals could you set for yourself that would enhance your life?**

JULY 7:
CONSISTENCY YIELDS RESULTS

When I was writing my doctoral dissertation, I created a calendar out of a large piece of poster board. I taped the calendar to the side of my refrigerator and every day I wrote down one task I would accomplish to get my research done. Each day I did that one task (more if I felt motivated but not less than that one task) and when I finished it, I wrote down a task for the next day. Sometimes the task was to read and summarize a research study. Other times it was simply to proofread a section I had already written. One day at a time, one task at a time, led me to finish my dissertation in record time. Consistent daily action was the secret to my doctoral success and it can be the secret to your weight loss success too. Thinness, permanent weight loss, comes from consistent daily action and not from abstinence or denial. If you focus on the habits you are trying to cultivate and practice them daily you will find that over time they sink in and you are on your way to permanent weight loss. I often say "it is what you do most of the time that creates results." Of the mindful eating habits you are learning, which ones are you practicing daily? Stick to them and the results you are seeking will come.

***Today:* Eat all your meals and snacks mindfully and meditate for twenty-five minutes.**

***Today's Journal Question:* What habits are you doing most of the time and what habits would you like to add into your daily routine?**

JULY 8:
HUNGER IS NOT AN EMERGENCY

As you are now well aware, tuning into your body's sensations of hunger is a key element of becoming a mindful eater. If you are like many of the people with whom I work, knowing what hunger is might have been somewhat foreign to you. You may have been so used to eating throughout the day (and maybe night) that you never really felt hungry. Or, at the first signs of hunger you immediately ate something, never giving your body a chance to fully express its need to eat. Over the years people have told me that they feared hunger. Among the reasons they offered was that they were afraid that if they let themselves get too hungry, they would eat too much. Some said they were afraid there would be no food when they needed it so they ate as soon as the first pang appeared. Feeling hunger (as we experience it in the

Western world) is not an emergency. It is not a call for immediate feeding.

Earlier I suggested that you measure your hunger using a Hunger Awareness Scale and choose to eat when you felt your hunger to be around a four or five. How are you doing with that? If you still find it hard to wait until you are at four or five on your scale, keep the idea that it's okay to feel hunger in mind. Be curious about your hunger instead of afraid of it. What does it feel like? Is it comfortable in any way? How long does it last? Typically, hunger will fade in about fifteen to twenty minutes without doing anything about it. If you are not at a four or five on your scale when you feel hunger, observe it and watch it fade. If it's too hard to watch it, distract yourself and see if twenty minutes later you notice it's gone. Waiting for the appropriate amount of hunger is skill. Not eating every time you feel a hunger pang is also a skill. Part of the reason why you may have been carrying extra weight could be a fear of being hungry. I hope by now you understand that hunger is a normal bodily function and nothing to fear. As far as I know, no one died from waiting fifteen minutes to eat.

***Today:* Eat all your meals and snacks mindfully and meditate for twenty-five minutes.**

***Today's Journal Question:* What would happen if you waited to eat when you initially feel hungry?**

JULY 9:
MINDFUL BITES, LICKS AND TASTES

Growing up one of my favorite things to do was to lick the spoon after my mother whipped up a batch of brownies or chocolate chip cookies. Back in the day we weren't warned about eating raw batter, so I didn't hesitate for a moment. Later when I started cooking for myself, I would taste-test my recipes along the way. A spoon full of tomato sauce to make sure it was salted properly. A strand of spaghetti to test for tenderness. A lick of frosting for good measure. Now that I understand mindfulness, I can see how much of that taste-testing was actually mindless eating. Truth be told, bites, licks and tastes were not limited to cooking time. I would bite, taste and lick my way through the day. I'm at lunch with a friend and she offers me a French fry, I take one. A colleague leaves some homegrown oranges with a note "help yourself," I do. These little bites, tastes and licks don't seem like much at the time but they are eating when not physically hungry. Since becoming a mindful eater, I mindfully choose whether to have bite, lick or taste when offered. Sometimes I do and other times I decline. Those times when I do accept, I make sure I am doing so with full attention. I no longer just pop the fry into my mouth. Now, I take a moment to experience its color, texture and scent. Then I savor it. I enjoy the fry so much more that way and can easily stop at one. If you indulge in bites, tastes and lick I encourage you to do so mindfully. I don't want to deny you the joy of a special treat; in fact, I want you to really enjoy it when offered. A mindful state of mind will yield maximum pleasure.

Today: **Eat all your meals and snacks mindfully and meditate for twenty-five minutes.**

Today's Journal Question: **Under what circumstances do you bite, taste, and lick?**

JULY 10:

MINDFUL CONSEQUENCES

One of the most significant contributions that mindfulness has made to my eating habits is becoming more aware of which foods work best for me and which ones do not. Before mindful eating, I ate what I thought I should, based on something that I read or heard. For example, when I started to feel the effects of perimenopause, I started drinking soy milk because I had read in a book about coping with menopause that this was a good idea. Within a few weeks of making this switch I was more miserable than before. I had more night sweats and hot flashes than I did when I wasn't drinking soy milk. For me, the suggestion to drink soy milk was NOT a good one! At the time I felt conflicted because the "experts" were telling me one thing and my body was screaming something else. Now that I am a mindful eater, I know to listen to my body and not the "experts." So, that means no more soy milk for me!

Becoming mindful of the consequences of the food you eat on your body will help you make better choices. Beginning today, pay attention to what foods and drinks do to your body. For example, does milk makes you gassy? Does sugar cause crashes? Does flour set up cravings? Does caffeine make it hard to sleep? Do tomatoes give you heartburn? If you suffer any of these symptoms, make the choice to not eat the foods that bother you. Being mindful of foods' consequences can also reveal which foods really work for you. For example, maybe you notice that having chicken in your salad fills you up and keeps you satisfied longer than beans do. This is great information to have, especially when you know that it will be a long time before your next meal or snack.

***Today:* Eat all your meals and snacks mindfully and meditate for twenty-five minutes.**

***Today's Journal Question:* Which foods work well with your body and which ones cause you discomfort, and could you mindfully choose to avoid those foods (or drinks) that hurt you and pick those that support your health and weight-loss goals?**

JULY 11:
PISTACHIO NUTS CAN TEACH YOU A LOT

Do like pistachios nuts? Those heart-healthy crunchy treats that peek through their hard shells, begging us to indulge? If you do, you can use them to learn more about mindful eating. Get yourself some pistachios in their shells. If you don't like pistachios, choose another shelled nut, such as walnuts. Not a nut fan; grab an orange. With shelled nuts or whole oranges, you have little choice but to be patient and eat slowly. The shells and peels are natural speed bumps. Enjoy a handful of nuts or a delectable orange mindfully. Engulf yourself with their aroma, feel and taste in doing so you will enjoy a most delicious mindful eating lesson.

***Today:* Eat all your meals and snacks mindfully and meditate for twenty-five minutes.**

***Today's Journal Question:* How does eating a food with a shell or peel affect how you eat it?**

JULY 12:
SHOW UP FOR YOURSELF

One of the more valuable things you can do for yourself is to show up. If you have a job, show up. If you have a parent-teacher conference, show up. If you have a dentist appointment, show up. Showing up is half the battle.

When you show up, you prove to yourself that you will do what you say you will do. After you show up and do what you need to do, you can let it go. It's no longer hanging around as an "I have to." Another way to show up is to show up for yourself. Show up when the only one watching is you. No boss. No teacher. No dentist. Just you. Let me give you an example from my own life. On a typical Sunday morning you can find me in a Zumba class. Zumba is a Latin-style dance class. Now let's be clear, I am not Latin and my body is not built to move to a Latin beat, but that doesn't stop me. I show up. I dance as best I can, glistening with sweat in my hot pink tank top. I may not look graceful and I certainly won't win any sparkling disco balls, but I go anyway. I show up for no one and no other reason than me. Showing up in this way fortifies my self-image as a person who takes care of herself as best she can. How do you show up for yourself?

***Today:* Eat all your meals and snacks mindfully and meditate for twenty-five minutes.**

***Today's Journal Question:* What can you do to show up for yourself?**

JULY 13:

EATING WITHOUT DISTRACTION, REALLY?

When people ask me for one tip to become a more mindful eater, I recommend that they eat without distraction. That means no TV, no phone, no book or computer, no driving, no working. Nothing. Just you and your food. Without distractions, a person can be more present with their food. More able to taste the flavors and know when they have had enough. Sounds good, right? It is. It's great advice. But it is impossible to eat completely without distraction because joining you as you eat is your chattering mind. Despite your best intentions, your mind will intrude on your meal. Thoughts of work, family, chores, you name it, will show up. You might want to focus on the taste of your bagel but your mind insists on rehashing yesterday's conversation with your co-worker. That's okay. Minds chatter. When your mind interrupts your meal, acknowledge it, thank it for its input and move your attention back to your food. Do this as many times as you need to. Eventually your mind will catch on and give you a break.

***Today:* Eat all your meals and snacks mindfully and meditate for twenty-five minutes.**

Today's Journal Question: **How does your chattering mind interfere with your mindful eating practices?**

JULY 14:
THE POWER TO CHOOSE

For me, the best part of mindful eating is the freedom to choose what and when to eat. There is such freedom knowing that I can go anywhere and do anything without being concerned about food. In my dieting days, when I didn't know better, I would stay home so I could eat what I was "supposed" to eat. The only times I would go out to dinner were those times when I was, shall we say, in between diets. I remember the feeling of freedom on those days when I could order whatever I wanted. Now, as a mindful eater, I feel that freedom daily. Because mindful eating gives us the power of choice over what and when to eat, we are free. Now when I am invited to dinner, I eagerly accept, knowing that as long as I check in with my hunger and fullness and keep the knowledge I gleaned from my Outer Guidance in mind, I am good to go anywhere at any time. With mindfulness is general, we always have the power to choose. When we practice mindfulness and are present in the here and now, we can choose what next action to take with full attention and focus. To me that's power. That's freedom.

Today: **Eat all your meals and snacks mindfully and meditate for twenty-five minutes.**

Today's Journal Question: **How will you exercise your power to choose today?**

JULY 15:
THE MINDFUL TRAVELER: SUPERMARKETS IN OTHER LANDS

As I have previously shared, I love to travel. I also told you that I love to photograph the foods I eat when I travel and even encouraged you to take a photo of your food before you eat it. What I also love to do when I travel is visit supermarkets. Well, maybe not a super market, but whatever markets local residents shop in. Whether I am in Shanghai or London, Nairobi or Phuket, I make it a point to see the markets. Some of the markets are outdoors and offer the freshest produce I have ever seen, and some produce I have never seen! It is amazing how much diversity there is in food depending upon where in the world you are or what time of year it is. Markets are like museums for me. I can wander for a long time, taking in the sights, smells and sounds. The good news is that you don't have to travel to get the experience of investigating other foods and cuisine. With a little Googling you can find lots of ethnic markets in your community. I recommend that you check them out. When we expand our horizons by exploring different foods, we help ourselves step out of the ruts of mindless eating we often fall prey to and learn to appreciate all the culinary wonders of the world. How marvelous!

***Today:* Eat all your meals and snacks mindfully and meditate for twenty-five minutes.**

***Today's Journal Question:* If you have ever explored a market in another country, what was your experience like?**

JULY 16:
BEING A MINDFUL EATER WHEN OTHERS ARE AROUND

If you are in the northern hemisphere, you are in the height of summer right now. And with summer comes barbecues, pool parties and beach picnics. And with summer barbecues, pool parties and beach picnics comes food. Lots and lots of food. What is a mindful eater to do when there is so much food to choose from and so many people around? Not knowing how to eat when you are with others is a common issue for new mindful eaters. When you are eating mindfully you may choose not to eat when others are eating because you are tuned into the fact that you are not hungry. Or as a mindful eater you may decide that you only want some of your favorite entrée and are not interested in any of the appetizers being served.

These are both good, mindful choices, but may be choices that might be unpopular with the other people around. In other words, eating mindfully may look different than the way you used to eat, the way people around you eat and the way the people around you expect you to eat and this could cause some challenges. I'd like to offer you two ideas for how to handle these kinds of situations. First, you could share your mindful eating lessons with the people around you. Educate them as to what you are doing and why. Tell them how mindful eating is changing your relationship to food and how it is guiding you to feel more peaceful around food and eating. Invite them to choose their favorite food and show them how to savor it. If this suggestion feels like TMI—too much information—you could take a different approach and say nothing about mindfulness and instead simply tell the people who are scrutinizing your eating that you are pacing yourself so you can enjoy the food more. As a mindful eater this is exactly what you are doing but you are not revealing the mindful nature of your actions up front. It has been my experience both personally and professionally that the people who pay attention to what, when and how much I eat have eating issues of their own and could do well to learn about mindful eating!

***Today:* Eat all your meals and snacks mindfully and meditate for twenty-five minutes.**

***Today's Journal Question:* How can you eat mindfully around people?**

JULY 17:
NATURAL PORTION CONTROL

An interesting thing happens as you continue to practice mindful eating—you become a natural portion controller. When I was first learning mindful eating, I either took too much food for my hunger or too little. It took a while for me to develop a sixth sense about exactly how much food I needed at any given moment. But eventually I did. Soon I could feel if the amount of food I was serving myself matched my hunger level. For example, I might be serving myself blueberries and after pouring some into my bowl, I would have this nagging feeling that there were too many. So, I would pick a few out. Then I would feel, nope—not enough, and toss two or three back into the bowl "knowing" I now had the right amount. I can't really explain it but I am confident you will understand what I am talking about soon enough. As a mindful eater, you get really tuned into your body and you learn exactly what and how much is right for you. As this knowing becomes second nature you naturally choose the right amount for you and without even realizing it are exercising natural portion control.

***Today:* Eat all your meals and snacks mindfully and meditate for twenty-five minutes.**

***Today's Journal Question:* Pay attention to how well you estimate how much food you need to eat at any given meal or snack and record your**

observations in your journal.

JULY 18:

SILENCING FOOD'S SIREN SONG

Back in June we explored foods that pull. Now, six weeks later, let's look at this topic again because it is a powerful one. Does food still talk to you? Does it still call your name? Are there still certain foods you find irresistible? Remember, many of us have foods that pull us in. We are pulled in physically in the form of cravings and we are pulled in psychologically by the promise of emotional well-being. In the beginning of becoming a mindful eater you may feel as if you spend a lot of time thinking about food and you are probably right. By going from mindless to mindful we are intentionally shifting our emphasis towards food. We are paying more attention to its taste and appearance, to its ability to satisfy or not.

When we first give ourselves permission to eat whatever foods we want, we may feel that pull more intensely. But over time, that pull fades away and foods that were important at one point are not so important anymore. The freedom that is inherent in mindful eating eliminates the pull. Is this starting to happen for you? As the emphasis on food at the beginning of the mindful eating process wears off, food's siren song silences and food takes its proper place in your life. If food is still pulling you, don't fret. Be curious about the why, what and when of the pull and use your mindful skills to understand it. If it is a food you really want, wait until the next time you are hungry and mindfully enjoy it.

***Today:* Eat all your meals and snacks mindfully and meditate for twenty-five minutes.**

***Today's Journal Question:* What foods pull you and why?**

JULY 19:

GOING FURTHER WITH OUTER GUIDANCE

Back in January, I first introduced you to the mindful eating tool of Outer Guidance. Since then, I have mentioned it from time to time. First, by using calories as a tool for making mindful decisions about what to eat. Later, I showed you how exercise can be a form of Outer Guidance and last month we explored Clean Eating as form of Outer Guidance. Beginning today, we will do more to cultivate your Outer Guidance so that you can become the architect of the most mindful selection of foods for you. During this coming week, experiment with three different forms of Outer Guidance to find the right foods for you. Perhaps you want to experiment with green smoothies to see how your body responds. If green is not your color, you could check out with healthy cooking techniques such as water-sautéing, poaching or broiling.

Not a cook? There are healthy meal delivery services where the food is delivery already prepared. Don't like to shop—how about getting fresh produce delivered to your door via a local co-op? The time has come for you to investigate for yourself the best nutritional information you can find for your particular needs. In the weeks and months to come, we will explore Outer Guidance as it relates to heart health and diabetes, organic and plant-based foods, and sugar, flour, dairy and caffeine products. But you don't have to wait for me. Begin your exploration today. Apply what you learn and keep track of the outcome. In no time at all you will be an expert in what foods are best for you.

Today: Eat all your meals and snacks mindfully and meditate for twenty-five minutes.

***Today's Journal Question:* What Outer Guidance will you seek out today?**

JULY 20:
OUTER GUIDANCE—GETTING THE FACTS

When following up on the importance of Outer Guidance and applying it to your eating choices, you may be asking, "How do I know if what I find is good information or junk science?" Great question! Here are some tips on how to tell if what you are learning about is reputable: (1) Determine where the data comes from. If it comes from a university, medical journal or documented study there may be merit to it. If it comes anecdotal stories or the researcher's personal experience, dig deeper. (2) What methodology was used to reach the conclusions offered? Double-blind studies are the gold standard in research, polling friends at a Super Bowl party not so much. (3) Are alternative theories explored, or is the only position offered that of the individual researcher? Not a good sign. (4) Is the research upon which the information is based replicable? In other words, if another scientist did the same research would they come up with the same results? Lastly, (5) is the information offered as revolutionary? As the old saying goes, "If it seems too good to be true, it probably is." If you decide that the Outer Guidance you found is in fact good science, the most reliable way for you to know if what you found is right for you is to test it. Apply the Outer Guidance and observe the results. If you feel good, you may be onto something. If you don't, move on and seek out more guidance elsewhere. One website I have come across that appears to offer trustworthy information is that of Dr. Michael Greger: NurtitionFacts.org. But don't take my word for it, check it out for yourself.

Today: **Eat all your meals and snacks mindfully and meditate for twenty-five minutes.**

Today's Journal Question: **How will you judge whether the Outer Guidance you come across is worth considering?**

JULY 21:
PRACTICE WITH MORE DIFFICULT FOOD

People tell me that it's easy to eat certain foods mindfully. For example, seldom is broccoli a struggle, or even chicken or fish. The trouble starts with food such as pasta, chocolate and french fries. I often hear laments about not being able to stop eating these foods once started. I understand. I felt that way about Starbucks' mochas. Truth be told, I didn't think I would ever be able to be mocha-free. There was a time when I thought life without a mocha would be unbearable. I used to think of it as my joy, the one high spot in an otherwise demanding day. I don't think that way anymore. Today I can have or not have a mocha and it makes no emotional difference. I am neutral about my mochas and I will tell you how I got here. I practiced. Today I will teach you how to practice with difficult foods so that you too can reach a point of take-it-or-leave-it. Remember back in January when we did the raisin experiment? You are going to do the same experiment with the foods that you find difficult. Here's what you do.

- Select a serving of food that challenges you. Let's use french fries as an example.
- Put the french fries onto a plate in front of you. Notice how you feel. You might feel excited, nervous, giddy or afraid. It doesn't matter. Just observe.
- Choose a french fry to start with and pick it up with your fingers. (If the food you chose to work with is not a finger food, then

place a small portion of it on a fork or spoon.)

- Look at it. Notice its colors and textures.
- Bring it to your nose and sniff. Notice its scent.
- Touch it to your lips. Feel its texture.
- Place it in your mouth, but don't chew. Feel it. Roll it over your tongue.
- Bite into it. Notice its flavor.
- Chew it but don't swallow.
- Now swallow and feel the food slip down your throat.
- Place your hand on your stomach and imagine the bite of food settling there.
- How do you feel?
- Repeat this process two or three more times and then stop.
- Notice how it feels to stop.
- Put the remaining french fries away. You can eat them again later if you wish.

When you practice mindful eating with difficult foods, you learn that you can be around them without overindulging. The more you practice with difficult foods, the more comfortable you become around them. As you learn that you can choose to have these difficult foods any time you are hungry, they lose their appeal.

***Today:* Eat all your meals and snacks mindfully and meditate for twenty-five minutes.**

***Today's Journal Question:* Make a list of foods you find difficult and practice eating them mindfully, making notes afterwards about your experience.**

JULY 22:
WHAT ARE YOUR EATING TRIGGERS?

By now you are probably pretty aware of the difference between physical and emotional hunger. Physical hunger is your body's cry for nourishment. Emotional hunger is your soul's cry for help. Some of the circumstances that lead to emotional eating maybe self-evident. You broke up with a romantic partner and you feel depressed so you eat. You get a huge bill in the mail and the anxiety over paying it sends you to the fridge. We call these circumstances emotional eating triggers. Some triggers are not so obvious and require a bit more introspection to discover. For example, when your back hurts, you eat. You are tired, so you eat. You spent the last month remodeling your house and you find yourself gaining weight. There are other subtle eating triggers including locations, like a movie theater where you always have popcorn. Or your favorite restaurant where you order your favorite dish because you don't eat it often. The easiest way for me to tell you how to identify eating triggers is to simply say, "Anytime you are eating when you are not physically hungry, you are responding to an eating trigger." It is important for you to master these eating triggers so you can stay on the mindful eating path. To get started, identify one situation that might act as an eating trigger. Carefully identify the thought, the emotion, and the physical response that accompanied that trigger and then explore how these three factors create the trigger that leads to your excess eating.

***Today:* Eat all your meals and snacks mindfully and meditate for twenty-five minutes.**

***Today's Journal Question:* What eating triggers can you identify?**

JULY 23:
"NOURISHMENT IS NOT JUST NUTRITION"

There is a passage in the book *Nourishing Wisdom* by Marc David that I love. It reads, "Nourishment is not just 'nutrition.' Nourishment is the nutrients in the food, the taste, the aroma, the ambiance of the room, the conversation at the table, the love and inspiration in the cooking, and the joy of the entire eating experience." While this book is not about mindful eating, I have yet to find a more beautiful description. I was so awed by these two sentences that I wrote them on a note card which I keep near my place setting. If I ever need reminding of what a mindful eating is, I read the card. I recommend you do the same. Write Marc's words down and keep them close. Before you eat, take a deep breath, get centered and read the card. Then, put your attention to each element: the nutrients, the taste, the smell, the sights, the sounds, and the love. Let it all soak in as you set an intention to enjoy your food.

***Today:* Eat all your meals and snacks mindfully and meditate for twenty-five minutes.**

Today's Journal Question: **Describe your reaction to the definition of nourishment above.**

JULY 24:
DEEPER DIVE INTO EMOTIONAL EATING

Three days ago, we began our exploration of eating triggers. Today I want to dive deeper into emotional eating because so much mindless eating is emotional. Recognizing the difference between emotional and physical hunger is paramount to changing your relationship with food. What is equally important is learning what to do when you feel emotionally hungry. The secret to getting a handle on emotional eating is having a set of go-to activities that can address the emotional need in the moment. Put another way, Step one is acknowledging that you are emotional hungry. Step two is identifying the emotion that is causing you to want to eat, and Step three is finding something else that will manage the emotion. For example, you live alone and weekends are often filled with chores and not much else. As a result, you find yourself filling your time with food. What's the emotion you are feeling that is causing you to eat? Probably loneliness. So, for Step three to work you need some ideas for what you can do to deal with your loneliness. Off the top of my head, I can think of four—date, find a hobby, make plans with friends, and volunteer. Each of these activities if done consistently can heal loneliness and end the emotional eating that goes with it.

Another example, you are in school, studying for final exams and taking snack breaks every hour. The emotion under the snacking is most likely anxiety. What go-to activities can you have in place to deal with your anxiety? The first one that comes to my mind is meditation. Maintaining your daily meditation practice can do wonders for a case of the jitters. Spend some time today brainstorming what activities can be your go-to activities to help you deal with your emotions without eating.

Today: **Eat all your meals and snacks mindfully and meditate for twenty-five minutes.**

Today's Journal Question: **Identify the top three emotions you eat over and list five go-to activities to cope with each.**

JULY 25:

CLEARING SPACE

Earlier this year we reviewed the mindfulness principle of letting go. Today I want to explore it again, but this time in terms of material goods. If you came into my home or office, you would notice that both places are neat. I am not a white glove kind of a person, but I do like things tidy. Having things in their place serves me well because I rarely misplace them. Having tidy surroundings does something else. It creates peace. Have you ever noticed that when you walk into a messy room you tense up? Or have you ever cleaned out a closet or drawer and felt a fabulous sense of relief? Uncluttering can even make you feel lighter. If you Google the words clutter and weight, you will find over thirty-three million hits reflecting books, articles, blogs, and websites devoted to the relationship between clutter and weight gain.

I haven't done the research, but I can tell you from my experience with clients, when they take control of their surroundings and let go of whatever is weighing them down in their environments, they start to lose weight. When we unclutter our homes, we simultaneously unclutter our body, mind and spirit. Look around you. Notice the condition of the places where you choose to live and work. What do they reflect? Are they packed and chaotic or open and serene? Spend some time over the next few weeks, uncluttering your environment. Let go of whatever no longer serves your best interest or highest good. Do this slowly. Pause and observe the items. Feel them in your hands. Remember where and when you got them. If they make you happy, keep them. If they don't, let them go. Create space in your home and your heart for whatever feels good to you and remove the rest. If you do this, you will very likely feel lighter in spirit and on the scale.

***Today:* Eat all your meals and snacks mindfully and meditate for twenty-five minutes.**

***Today's Journal Question:* What can you let go of today?**

JULY 26:

THE SOUNDS AROUND US

For some reason I can't explain, two of my neighbors have decided to remodel their homes at the same time. For the past week, each morning as I sit for my meditation practice, I am serenaded by jackhammering and pounding. One sound coming from the left, the other from the right. I could be annoyed, frustrated, angry, but instead I choose to practice equanimity ("it is what it is") and I sit down. On those mornings I use the noise from the construction as the focus of my meditation. Instead of directing myself back to my breath when my mind wanders, I direct myself back to the sounds. Suddenly, they are no longer noise. Rather, they are the musical refrain of my day. Because I am paying attention, I notice the rhythm of the hammering and the beat of the pounding. They are no longer clamor. They are music. When they stop, I am aware of the stillness and the silence that prevails. Truth be told I have been enjoying my practice this week. Don't tell anyone but I will miss them when they are gone. If sounds show up while you are meditating, incorporate them into your practice. Whether it is a horn, siren or baby's cry, they are part of life and can be celebrated as such.

***Today:* Eat all your meals and snacks mindfully and meditate for twenty-five minutes.**

***Today's Journal Question:* What sounds are in your environment which you can incorporate into your meditation practice?**

JULY 27:

A GRATEFUL MIND DOESN'T EAT

I once heard it said that a grateful mind doesn't eat. I thought about that remark and came to agree with it. I have done quite a bit of reading on the psychology of gratitude and often recommend it to my clients as a tool for personal growth. Among the benefits of a regular gratitude practice is improved mood. This is especially valuable if you eat in response to a bad mood. There are many ways to practice gratitude. Here are some of my favorites: (1) keep a daily gratitude journal and each day write about something or someone you are grateful for and why; (2) send thank you notes to people who have done something you appreciate; (3) express gratitude for your food before you eat; (4) write "thank you" on the memo lines of checks you send out or on the back of checks you endorse; and (5) express gratitude for yourself each night before you go to sleep by acknowledging something you did well or good during the day. Cultivating an attitude of gratitude is one of the healthiest mindful habits you can develop. See what happens in your life when you are grateful.

***Today:* Eat all your meals and snacks mindfully and meditate for twenty-five minutes.**

***Today's Journal Question:* How might practicing gratitude improve your mindful eating habits?**

JULY 28:

MY BODY—HOW ART THOU?

Do you live from the neck up? So many people I have worked with over the years tell me that they don't look at or know their body. Their face they see, but they avoid everything else. Is that true for you, too? With mindful eating we try to bring more attention to the body both in regard to physical hunger and to other experiences, as well as to how feelings and emotions are experienced. If you are out of touch with your body, I would like to invite you make friends with it. Regardless of how you may look, your body is a precious gift. Take time to recognize what is good about your body. Do you have arms that can carry a crying child? Do you have legs that can dance at a friend's wedding? Do you have eyes that can admire a sunrise or ears that can hear a symphony? Try to balance whatever is unappealing to you about your body with positive appreciation and acceptance for all your body does for you.

***Today:* Eat all your meals and snacks mindfully and meditate for twenty-five minutes.**

***Today's Journal Question:* How can you get to know and appreciate your body better?**

JULY 29:

FOOD—FRIEND OR FOE?

You are more than halfway into your year's journey with me. So, I'd like to know how your attitude towards food has changed so far. Is food a friend or enemy? Are you more comfortable around food? Are there foods you can now take or leave? Think back to which foods are challenging for you and consider if they still are. My hope is that by now your relationship to food and eating has shifted and you are feeling more peaceful. If you are still struggling, no worries. Take some time to reflect on what attempts you have been making and what might be holding you back. For instance, are you getting good at noticing your physical hunger but not so sure when you are full?

Or maybe you know when you are full but can't quite get up from the table with food on your plate. Give yourself a pat on the back for what you have been doing and show yourself some compassion for where you are having trouble. Your journey will progress further if you give extra attention to the basics. Michael Jordan, one of the greatest basketball players of all time, has said, "Get the fundamentals down and the level of everything else will rise." This is a man who credits his success to hours spent shooting baskets and performing basic drills. You would think that at his level he wouldn't have had to do that, but he knew that the stronger the foundation the better the results. Practice your mindful eating fundamentals and you will get to the point where you are at peace with food.

***Today:* Eat all your meals and snacks mindfully and meditate for twenty-five minutes.**

***Today's Journal Question:* How has your attitude towards food changed so far?**

JULY 30:

SWIPE RIGHT/SWIPE LEFT

In today's dating world, singles are swiping right and swiping left to meet their mates. In the world of meditation, we are also interested in rights and lefts but in particular, the right and left hemispheres of the brain. Neuroscience teaches us that the frontal cortex of our brains affects how we feel. To simplify, the right frontal cortex is where depression lives and the left frontal cortex is where happiness lives. Research has revealed that meditation changes the structure of the brain. Specifically, meditation shifts brain activity from right to left, from depression to happiness. This helps explain why we feel better after we have cultivated a meditation practice. Pay attention to how your mood changes as a result of an established meditation practice.

***Today:* Eat all your meals and snacks mindfully and meditate for twenty-five minutes.**

***Today's Journal Question:* How has your meditation practice affected your moods?**

JULY 31:

THOUGHT—PAUSE—RESPOND

Applying mindfulness to every aspect of our lives can be very rewarding. Learning to be more aware of our moment-to-moment existence can make life richer. If you are still struggling with what this means and how to do it, I'd like to share with you a simple technique to help you along. I call it "Thought—Pause—Respond." This technique creates a space between a thought and a reaction. Without that space we are on auto-pilot merely reacting as we always have without any consideration of current circumstances. It is within that space that life happens. If you ever studied psychology, you may be familiar with the work of Pavlov and his dogs.

Pavlov discovered that dogs automatically salivate when presented with food. When he offered the dogs food at the same time as he rang a bell, the dogs learned to salivate to the sound of the bell whether there was food available or not. The dogs developed a conditioned response to the bell. Sorry to say, but we are all Pavlov's dogs! We are all conditioned to respond automatically to situations with which are familiar. This is especially true when it comes to food and drink. We have learned to eat in response to stimuli (aka thoughts) that have nothing to do with food. To break this pattern, or any other automatic behavior, simply take a pause between the stimulus (the thought) and your response. This pause creates the space in which you can now choose how to respond, whether it's to a thought about eating something, a comment made by a coworker or the sunset you see on your ride home from work.

***Today:* Eat all your meals and snacks mindfully and meditate for twenty-five minutes.**

***Today's Journal Question:* Practice "Thought—Pause—Respond" and reflect on your experience in your journal.**

AUGUST

◆◆◆

AUGUST 1:

THIRTY-MINUTE MEDITATION BUMP UP

It's time to once again bump up your meditation practice. This time we are expanding to thirty minutes. Thirty minutes will be the length of time we will stay at for the remainder of our journey. If you feel ready to extend your sitting time, start today. If not stay where you are and add minutes at a pace that suits you. When you are ready for a thirty-minute meditation session, set your timer for thirty minutes and give it a try. Remember, if you are not ready for this bump, no worries. That's okay.

Acknowledge yourself for what you have done to date. If you are still not doing any meditation at all, why not? What is stopping you? Time? Anxiety? Investigate what is getting in your way. Be curious about your challenge. What is it all about? What would help you break through? Be patient and gentle with yourself. Question what is happening from a position of non-judgment and self-compassion. Remember, if you are really struggling, consider attending a meditation class as I recommended before. Sitting with others maybe exactly what you need to get going with your practice.

***Today:* Eat all your meals and snacks mindfully and meditate for thirty minutes.**

***Today's Journal Question:* How do you feel about increasing your meditation time to thirty minutes?**

AUGUST 2:

WHO ARE YOU?

When you meet a new person is one the first questions you ask, "What do you do?" Typically it is, and typically we define ourselves by our work. I'm a psychologist. You are a teacher. He's a banker. She's a doctor. We also identify ourselves by who we are in relationship to others. I am a daughter. You are a wife. She is a mother. He is an uncle. But we are so much more than how we earn a paycheck and who we spend time with. We are each unique, multi-dimensional creatures with individual personalities and identities, and yet, when asked, "Who are you?" we may find it hard to answer. Self-identity is based on self-perception and self-perception is how you see yourself. I once heard it said if you want to know who you really are, observe yourself when no one is looking.

In other words, watch your behavior to find out who you are. Think about your behavior around food. Your behavior defines you. If you want to make changes in how you live, you need to make changes in your identity. You need a new identity based on the new behavior. "Becoming a mindful eater" is a new identity. "I eat when I'm hungry and I stop when I am full" is a new identity. "I don't emotionally eat" is a new identity. "I am a meditator" is a new identity. Decide for yourself what you would like your new identity to be and then act on it. Practice the behaviors that are consistent with your desired identity and soon you will become that identity. You have to change who you are to make permanent changes; any less is temporary.

***Today:* Eat all your meals and snacks mindfully and meditate for thirty minutes.**

***Today's Journal Question:* Who are you and is it who you want to be?**

AUGUST 3:
FALLING IN LOVE WITH THE ORDINARY

When you apply mindfulness to the everyday events in your life, you experience them more deeply. An orange is more than an orange when you stop to caress its texture, inhale its aroma, and savor its sweetness. An airplane flight is more than transportation when you hear the hum of the engine, feel the lift as you get airborne and take in the panoramic view of the earth outside your window. Mindfulness lets you fall in love with the ordinary. In fact, the ordinary stops being ordinary and become extraordinary when you notice it. Each moment is unique. Each person, blade of grass and event is special if you let it be. For today, notice the extraordinary within the ordinary. See if you can find the fullness, uniqueness and specialness of your everyday life. See if you can fall in love with the ordinary.

***Today:* Eat all your meals and snacks mindfully and meditate for thirty minutes.**

***Today's Journal Question:* What ordinary event of the day became extraordinary when you paid mindful attention to it?**

AUGUST 4:
A HISTORY LESSON

Our history books are filled with tales of adventure, conflict and triumphs. But what about food? What is the history of food? Did you know that legend tells us the chocolate chip cookie was made by accident after a restauranteur tried to make chocolate batter and the chocolate morsels never melted? Or that peas are the world's oldest known vegetable? Are you curious about where cauliflower comes from? Or what people ate in Colonial America? Food is fascinating when you pay attention to it. Instead of being mindless about the origins of your next meal, do some research.

For example, this morning I had yogurt for breakfast. I googled yogurt and learned that it came into being in Central Asia around 6000 B.C. It was at this time that Neolithic herdsman began milking their animals and the enzymes in the pouches where they carried the milk caused it to curdle and form yogurt. Who knew? All of a sudden, my morning breakfast became much more interesting. Exploring the origins of the food we eat focuses our attention on it. We become more connected to it and as a result more mindful. How much do you know about the food you eat? Are you curious?

***Today:* Eat all your meals and snacks mindfully and meditate for thirty minutes.**

***Today's Journal Question:* Research the origins of a food you typically eat and record what you discover.**

AUGUST 5:
TRY A NEW FRUIT OR VEGETABLE

Are you in a food rut? It's easy to slip into one so if you are, don't feel bad. Most of us have our standards which we rely on day in and day out. Today I'd like you to try something new. Branch out. The easiest way to do that is with fruits and vegetables. There are so many to choose from and yet most of us simply go for the ordinary—apples, bananas and berries or carrots, tomatoes, and lettuce. Even within our ordinary selections there is enormous variety. Have you ever eaten a green apple instead of a red one? How about a plantain instead of a "regular" banana? Boysenberries instead of blueberries? Heirloom tomatoes instead of cherry? White carrots instead of orange ones? Or butter leaf lettuce rather than romaine? Choosing the same foods over and over again is a form of mindlessness and since our goal is to become more mindful, try a new fruit or vegetable today. Not sure how to do that, ask your local grocer. Go to the produce section of your favorite store and ask one of the employees for a recommendation. If you shop at a farmer's market, talk to the farmers and get their suggestions. Make your section and eat it mindfully. If it requires cooking, cook it with your full attention and admiration. If you can simply bite into to it, find a peaceful spot and savor it. Notice how it feels to do something different. Are you enjoying the flavor and texture of your choice? Could it become a regular food for you? If you don't like it, why not? Make a game out of trying new foods regularly. Maybe once a week or once a month you can try something new. What have you got to lose?

Today: **Eat all your meals and snacks mindfully and meditate for thirty minutes.**

Today's Journal Question: **Try a new fruit or vegetable today and document your experience.**

AUGUST 6:

NATURALLY THIN INTERVIEW

There is a myth circulating among dieters that naturally thin people can eat anything and everything whenever they want in whatever quantities they want without gaining an ounce. There may be some for whom this might be true, for example teenage boys during a growth spurt, but for the rest of us mere mortals this idea is simply false. The naturally thin people I know work at it. They are mindful without even knowing they are. They think about their food choices. They watch their portion sizes. They use "treats" as "treats," not everyday indulgences. Don't agree? Okay, do an experiment. Interview three or four people you think are naturally thin or who have healthy eating patterns and healthy weights.

Specifically, ask these people the following questions: (1) how do they choose what to eat; (2) how much to eat; (3) and when to eat; (4) how do they decide to stop; (5) how do they decide to eat a favorite food and how do they stop when they do; (6) do they eat snacks, if yes, what kind of snacks and how often; (7) ask them if they ever overeat and what overeating means to them. If you don't want to ask these kinds of questions, simply observe them. Watch as they make food choices. See who leaves food on their plate. Listen for who talks about being hungry or full. Go shopping with them and notice what they people put in their grocery carts? Review your findings and decide which of their habits you might like to add to your habits, then practice them.

***Today:* Eat all your meals and snacks mindfully and meditate for thirty minutes.**

***Today's Journal Question:* How do the naturally thin people in your life eat?**

AUGUST 7:
FORBIDDEN FRUIT

I am sure you know by now, it can be easy to stay mindful when you are eating food that is "okay" to eat. You know what I mean—broccoli, chicken, salad. But what about the food you believe is not okay to eat? Early on I explained that with mindful eating, no food is off limits. There are no food lists or legal vs illegal foods. There are no red light or green light foods. Foods are equal and you choose what to eat based on your body's needs and preferences. So, I have a question for you. Have you made all food equal or are there still foods that you stay away from because you fear them? Have you been practicing eating difficult food mindfully? Or are you still afraid you won't be able to stop when you are full or that they will trigger a binge? To truly make all foods equal I would like you to practice eating those forbidden ones. Pick a food that you avoid and do the following exercise. Repeat this exercise as many times you want to with as many foods as you need to until you truly embrace the idea of equal foods. Here are the instructions. They will be familiar to you.

- Choose your forbidden food and place it on a beautiful plate or bowl.
- Sit quietly in front of your food and take several deep breaths.
- Look closely at the food you have chosen and notice if any negative thoughts or feeling arise.
- If such thoughts or feelings are present, acknowledge them without judgment.
- Pick up a bite or piece of your forbidden food and notice its col-

ors and textures. Bring it to your nose and notice its scent. Touch the food to your lips and feel its texture.

- Place the food in your mouth, but don't chew. Feel it. Roll it over your tongue.
- When you are ready, bite into it. Chew it but don't swallow. Notice its flavor.
- Now swallow and feel the food slip down your throat.
- Place your hand on your stomach and imagine the bite of food settling there.
- Repeat this process with several more bites.
- With each bite, notice any thoughts or feelings that surface.
- Pay attention to the food's taste and ask yourself if it is as good as you expected. If it is, savor it. If it is not, you might choose to stop eating.
- Finish eating your portion and sit for a moment reflecting on the experience.
- Has your opinion of the food or your ability to eat changed?
- Keep practicing until you know you can eat this food mindfully.

Today: **Eat all your meals and snacks mindfully and meditate for thirty minutes.**

Today's Journal Question: **What forbidden food would you like to eat mindfully today?**

AUGUST 8:

YOGA AND MINDFUL MOVEMENT

Today we are going to add movement to your routine. Not exercise for weight loss but rather mindful movement where you are in touch with your body and its grace. One way to add mindful movement is to do yoga. If you already have a yoga practice, enjoy a session today. If you do not currently practice yoga, you might want to consider trying it. Many yoga studios offer a free introductory lesson. Check it out. Or you can find some videos online and see if you like it. If yoga is not your thing, then you can try walking or dance. Any activity can be done mindfully if it is done with intention and focus. Do whatever activity you choose slowly and deliberately. Feel your body move in space. Notice how it feels when it touches a surface. Be present in your body and enjoy its wonders.

***Today:* Eat all your meals and snacks mindfully, meditate for thirty minutes and move mindfully for ten minutes.**

***Today's Journal Question:* How can you incorporate mindful movement into your life?**

AUGUST 9:

ARE YOU YOUR OWN JUDGE, JURY AND EXECUTIONER?

It is so easy to be hard on ourselves, to expect more from ourselves than we expect from others. Does this describe you? Mindfulness can help soften your relationship with yourself. The mindful skill that does this is called self-compassion. Dr. Kristen Neff, author of the book titled *Self-Compassion*, suggests that you write a letter to yourself from the most compassionate version of yourself. In this letter, let your most compassionate self offer you love, comfort, guidance and support. Use your imagination to fill the letter with everything you would ever want to read to make yourself feel better. After you have finished the letter, put it away and save it for later. Pull it out and read it anytime you are being your own worst critic.

***Today:* Eat all your meals and snacks mindfully, meditate for thirty minutes and move mindfully for ten minutes.**

***Today's Journal Question:* What are the most compassionate words you can offer yourself?**

AUGUST 10:

CONTINUITY AND REPETITION ARE KEY

In graduate school, I took a course called *Theories of Learning*. This course offered ways to understand how we learn. Later, as a professor, I taught my students these theories of learning and urged them to use what I taught to get good grades in my class. Want to know that secret to learning? It's continuous repetition. It is through repetition that we learn everything—the good stuff and the not so good; good habits and bad ones. Every time you floss your teeth you are learning to floss your teeth daily. Every time you reach for candy after a bad day you are learning to use food to cope and every time you eat without distraction you are learning mindful eating.

Since January, I have been encouraging you to repeat the new (good) habits that form the foundation of a lifetime of mindful eating and healthy weight management. Today I want to remind you to continue practicing them. What am I taking about? You know: Continuing to being aware of the difference between physical hunger cues and emotional or other triggers to eat; assessing your level of hunger and fullness; sitting for your daily meditation practice; and using mindfulness in your everyday life. The more you repeat these actions the more quickly they become second nature.

***Today:* Eat all your meals and snacks mindfully, meditate for thirty minutes and move mindfully for ten minutes.**

***Today's Journal Question:* How have you been doing with repetitive learning?**

AUGUST 11:
ARE YOU RESISTANT TO EATING LESS?

One of the reasons why people lose weight when they become mindful eaters is that they eat smaller portions. These smaller portions come about not because they weigh and measure what they eat or because they limit themselves. Rather, these smaller portions are the result of listening to their Inner Wisdom and eating exactly what their body needs. Our culture is so used to oversized servings that when we eat according to our bodies' needs, we eat much less. One complaint I hear often is that people don't want to eat less.

They are disappointed that their portion sizes are shrinking. They are happy their waist size is shrinking but they want their food! Do you feel this way? Are you resistant to eating less food? If you are, it may be because you are still using food to assuage emotional pain. When you find yourself wanting to eat more than what your body is asking for, pause, take a deep breath, put your hand on your stomach and ask yourself, *why do you want to eat more than you need?* Listen for the answer. Then, make a mindful decision on how to proceed. If you want to keep eating, eat with full awareness. If you want to do something else, go for it. And, remember, if you follow your Inner Wisdom, you will be hungry again and you can eat again later.

***Today:* Eat all your meals and snacks mindfully, meditate for thirty minutes and move mindfully for ten minutes.**

***Today's Journal Question:* How do you feel about listening to your body and perhaps eating smaller portions than you used to?**

AUGUST 12:

DON'T JUDGE OTHERS WHEN THEY EAT MINDLESSLY

Throughout this journey we have explored the principle of non-judgment and how important is to not judge ourselves or our foods. It is equally important not to judge others, especially when we see them eating mindlessly. You know by now how easy it is to eat mindlessly. Our entire society is set up for that very endeavor. With food everywhere and with eating acceptable everywhere, you will be surrounded by mindless eaters. Please resist the temptation to comment on their eating. I know you know the benefits of mindful eating and how taking a mindful approach has enhanced your life and can appreciate that you might want to spread the word. The best way to spread the word is by example. People will start to notice the changes in you and that is the time to mention that you are a mindful eater. People need to come to mindful eating on their own. Changing a lifetime of habits is hard work and you can't make anyone do it if they don't want to. Instead, do as Mahatma Gandhi famously said, "Be the change that you wish to see in the world."

***Today:* Eat all your meals and snacks mindfully, meditate for thirty minutes and move mindfully for ten minutes.**

***Today's Journal Question:* How can you demonstrate mindful eating to those around you without judging them on their current eating habits?**

AUGUST 13:

WHAT RESISTS REALLY DOES PERSIST

There is an expression you may have heard—"what resists persists." To get rid of whatever is persisting, you need acceptance not resistance.

Acceptance is the opposite of resistance. When you accept what is instead of demanding what isn't, you find relief. In that relief you may find peace and whatever was bothering you may not be a bother anymore at all. I am sure you can guess where I am going with this. Mindfulness, which has been our focus all year long, is the skill that teaches us to accept rather than resist whatever is present. With mindfulness we deal with what is, not with what we wish was. We learn to accept reality but keep in mind, acceptance is not resignation. Acceptance, it turns out, is a powerful position that leads to transformation. Once we accept what is we can go about changing it, not through brute force but rather through compassion, kindness and patience. When you let go of the rope, the tug-of-war ends.

***Today:* Eat all your meals and snacks mindfully, meditate for thirty minutes and move mindfully for ten minutes.**

***Today's Journal Question:* What part of this process to mindful eating are you resisting?**

AUGUST 14:

BOOTS ON THE GROUND

Here's a trick you can use whenever you feel "off," whenever you feel as if anxiety is getting the best of you or you feel as if you are losing yourself to overwhelm. Put both feet on the ground. That's right, both of them. Toes, balls, soles and heels. In shoes or without, sitting or standing, doesn't matter. Now feel the ground. Focus your attention on the sensations of your feet touching the floor. Rock your feet back and forth noticing each time they make contact with the floor. If you like, stand up and feel the weight of your body and your feet on the ground.

Next, notice the moment. Where are you right now? What do you see around you, right now? What do you hear? Smell? Be present in this moment. Right now. Right here. Remind yourself that right now, in this moment, with your feet firmly on the ground, you are fine. Everything is okay. Right now, all is well. If your mind wanders to the future or replays the past, press your feet on to the ground and repeat, right here, right now, all is well. Repeat that phrase as many times as you need to, until you feel centered. Once centered, go on with your day.

***Today:* Eat all your meals and snacks mindfully, meditate for thirty minutes and move mindfully for ten minutes.**

***Today's Journal Question:* How can getting centered by putting your feet firmly on the ground get you through some tough moments?**

AUGUST 15:
BEEP TO BREATH

Do you hold your breath? I don't mean when you are diving into a pool. I mean while you are going about your ordinary business. Many of us do. If we are not holding our breath we are certainly breathing shallowly from our chest. Breathing more deeply has many health benefits including less stress, lower blood pressure, fewer aches and pains and better sleep. Getting into the habit of deep breathing is easy with this little tip. Set a timer to beep periodically throughout the day. When you hear the beep, take three deep breaths, and go on with your day. You can set the timer to beep as often as you like. It's up to you. I think you will find that with these little breathing breaks, you get energized and more focused. The more you do it, the better you will feel.

***Today:* Eat all your meals and snacks mindfully, meditate for thirty minutes and move mindfully for ten minutes.**

***Today's Journal Question:* Set your timer today and before you go to sleep, describe how taking these breathing breaks affected your day.**

AUGUST 16:
PRACTICING WEIGHT MANAGEMENT

Getting to and staying at the weight you want is all about maintaining the lifestyle habits that support that weight. Before you began learning mindful eating, your habits of mindless and emotional eating, yo-yoing on and off diets and intermittent bursts of exercise maintained your former weight. The habits that will support your new weight are the habits you have been practicing for the last seven months—meditation, noticing your hunger and fullness levels, savoring your food instead of rushing through your meals, and coping with your emotions in more effective ways. Just like concert pianists and world-class athletes continue to practice even when they have achieved greatness, you too need to keep practicing your mindful skills. Keep doing what you have been doing, bring it up a notch where you may be slacking and your new habits will take you to and keep you where you want to be.

Today: **Eat all your meals and snacks mindfully, meditate for thirty minutes and move mindfully for ten minutes.**

Today's Journal Question: **What habits have you been cultivating that are creating the changes you want and what habits need some improving?**

AUGUST 17:

OUTER GUIDANCE—HEART HEALTH

We use Outer Guidance in mindful eating as a tool to inform our decisions about what and when to eat. Some people are eager to address health concerns using food and I support that idea, if they do so mindfully. Blindly following a "heart-healthy diet" may not be what is exactly right for your body. Working alongside your physician, mindfully adopt nutritional suggestions and assess how your body responds. Experiment with one suggestion at a time and check in with yourself to see how you feel and what benefits you derive. It may seem easier to use a one-size-fits all approach but if you choose to address your heart health one mindful idea at a time, in the end you will have created an approach that uniquely suits your body.

Today: **Eat all your meals and snacks mindfully, meditate for thirty minutes and move mindfully for ten minutes.**

Today's Journal Question: **If a healthy heart is something you would like to achieve, what nutritional suggestion can you mindfully test today?**

AUGUST 18:

NURTURING JOY

If you are like many people, myself included, food is associated with joy. For example, family dinners filled with laughter, plastic pumpkins overflowing with candy, heart-shaped chocolates on Valentine's Day, gooey Easter eggs in a basket. These associations are powerful and are—and should continue to be—an important part of your life. The problem becomes when the food itself is the source of joy. When eating provides you pleasure because nothing else will. It's the carton of ice cream you eat while in your pjs on the couch watching reruns of *The Real Housewives*. It's the drive-thru meal that you allow yourself "because you deserve some fun." It's looking to food to bring happiness into your life even if only for a moment.

Instead of doing that, let's look at how you can bring joy into your life in other ways. I call this "Nurturing Joy." Deliberately, mindfully invite joyful events into your life. Seek them out the way you would seek out food for a binge. So, what are joyful events? For me they include: a walk along the beach feeling the ocean swirl around my ankles; holding a baby or small child; singing Frank Sinatra songs with friends while playing Scrabble; and bringing home a fresh bouquet of flowers from the farmer's market. As you go through the day notice the moments where you might feel a tinge of joy. See if you can add more of them over time. By nurturing joy in this way, you may find that you are less drawn to seeking joy through food.

Today: **Eat all your meals and snacks mindfully, meditate for thirty minutes and move mindfully for ten minutes.**

Today's Journal Question: **What are joyful events you can invite into your life to nourish joy?**

AUGUST 19:
HOPEFULNESS CHECK-IN

You are more than halfway through your journey to learning mindful eating, so I want to do a hopefulness check-in. Think about these questions: (1) Since being introduced to mindful eating, do you believe that it is possible to lose weight and make peace with food without dieting? (2) In this journey, have you discovered other ways to deal with emotional hunger other than eating? (3) As a result of mindfulness, are you eating emotionally less often? (4) Is your meditation practice making a difference in how reactive you are to life events? and (5) Are you looking forward to what the rest of the year's journey will bring? My hope is that you answered "yes" to all these questions and you are feeling hopeful about good things to come. If you answered "no" to any of the questions, go back and revisit these topics again.

Today: **Eat all your meals and snacks mindfully, meditate for thirty minutes and move mindfully for ten minutes.**

Today's Journal Question: **After considering the questions above, how hopeful are you that this journey can get you where you want to go?**

AUGUST 20:
WHY ARE YOU OUT OF BALANCE?

By paying more attention to your food, your eating habits and your life in general, you may notice that things are out of balance. For instance, by being more mindful of your day-to-day activities you may have noticed that you spend more time at work than you would like to. Or you may have noticed that you eat more fruits and vegetables on the weekend than during the week. Or, perhaps, your social life is nonexistent. Being out of balance is a common phenomenon and one that you can correct. The key is to notice where the imbalances lay and then get creative about restoring the balance. Spend too much time at work? Maybe you can telecommute one day a week. Not eating enough fruit during the week? Carry apples and bananas with you for a mindful snack. No social life? Join a club and make some friends. When we apply mindfulness to all aspects of our lives, we can find what works and what needs some attention.

Today: **Eat all your meals and snacks mindfully, meditate for thirty minutes and move mindfully for ten minutes.**

Today's Journal Question: **What in your life needs rebalancing and what are you going to do about it?**

AUGUST 21:
WHAT'S GOING RIGHT?

I have spent most of my professional life seeing clients as a clinical psychologist. Most people come into therapy because they are in pain and the majority of their therapy time is spent focused on what is wrong. Of course, it is important to look at the causes of one's pain, but it is equally important to focus our attention on what is going right. It is easy to get stuck in the disappointments, regrets and trauma of our lives and to feel, as a consequence, that nothing will ever get better. When we are mired in sorrow, we lose sight of or forget what went well, what has healed, and what is improving. Part of being mindful is to be present with all parts of ourselves and our lives—the positive and the negative; to experience the bad without judgment or recrimination, and to allow the good stuff to get their acknowledgments. Today, when your mind wanders to the negative intentionally shift your attention to something positive. Having a bad day at work, think of the great parking spot you got when you arrived. Remembering the fight you had with a friend last night, think about the friend you shared a laugh with today. With mindful attention you can train your mind to see what is going right in your life, not just what is going awry.

***Today:* Eat all your meals and snacks mindfully, meditate for thirty minutes and move mindfully for ten minutes.**

***Today's Journal Question:* What went right for you today?**

AUGUST 22:

IT'S ALL RIGHT!

I discovered a mantra, affirmation, prayer, call it what you wish, that helped me as I moved along my mindful eating path. Before each meal or snack, after I centered myself, spent a few moments getting in touch with my Inner Wisdom, and took a few deep breaths, I would say to myself, "This is the right food, in the right amount, for my body, right now." Repeating this short sentence assured me that I am okay, and my choices are okay. This sentence had a calming effect on me and led to greater satisfaction and often smaller portions because I was so tuned into my Inner Wisdom. To this day, I repeat this reassuring statement to myself often. It is working for me; maybe it will work for you too.

***Today:* Eat all your meals and snacks mindfully, meditate for thirty minutes and move mindfully for ten minutes.**

***Today's Journal Question:* For a few times today, try saying, "This is the right food, in the right amount, for my body, right now" before you eat or drink something. Reflect on that experience in your journal.**

AUGUST 23:

IS TV YOUR MEDICINE?

Did you know that TV watching can lead to weight gain? When we watch TV, we are typically sitting around being inactive. We may even be eating while we watch as a way to comfort ourselves or alleviate boredom. In addition, our food choices can be influenced by what we see on TV. Burgers dripping with cheese and bacon. Beautiful people indulging in decadent ice cream bars. Sports fans gathering around a table of chips and dips. These images and the emotions they evoke can influence our food choices if we are not mindful.

Now don't get me wrong, I love TV. I have many favorite shows that I hate to miss. Watching TV can be a source of joy when we do so mindfully. When watching TV, just watch TV, no mindless eating. Also, be mindful of how much time you spend watching TV and notice if you are using TV to avoid tasks or situations. Ask yourself if this is really how you want to spend your life or is there something else you might like to do? Maybe it's time to join a tennis league? If you have emotional issues you are ignoring by focusing your attention on TV maybe it's time for some therapy sessions? Think about the role TV plays in your life and how much or your TV viewing is mindless.

Today: **Eat all your meals and snacks mindfully, meditate for thirty minutes and move mindfully for ten minutes.**

Today's Journal Question: **In what way is TV watching a factor in your weight issues?**

AUGUST 24:

OUTER GUIDANCE: PLANT-BASED FOODS

On my journey to becoming a mindful eater I spent a lot of time reading books about the value of plant-based foods. I knew that fruits and vegetables are important because my mother told me so, and mother is always right! Growing up we traditionally had a salad with dinner (it was mostly iceberg lettuce, but it counted), while as an adult, with an extremely busy life, I found it hard to find time to make a salad. (As I write these words for you, I am chuckling to myself. Really, Sheila? No time to make a salad? Busted!)

As I ventured more into the science behind plant-based diets and the value of eating more plant-based foods, I used that knowledge to inform my choices. When dining out, I would often choose a salad entrée instead of something else. Not because I "should" eat the salad, but because I was learning that for me, for my body, eating more raw vegetables was a good thing. Choosing plant-based foods does not mean going vegan, or even vegetarian, it simply means eating more fruits, vegetables, whole grains, nuts and seeds. Experiment for yourself to see how adding various plant-based foods work for you. As author Michael Pollan famously said, "Eat food. Not too much. Mostly plants." Mindfully add some of these foods to your repertoire and see what happens.

Today: **Eat all your meals and snacks mindfully, meditate for thirty min-**

utes and move mindfully for ten minutes.

Today's Journal Question: **If you were to add more plant-based foods to your food choices, which foods would you like to add?**

AUGUST 25:
A DIFFERENT KIND OF FAST

Have you ever fasted to lose weight? Fasting as a diet trend shows up once in a while. There are medical as well as religious reasons to fast, but as general approach to weight management I can't recommend it. I would, however, like to recommend a different kind of fast. A fast that will support your mindfulness practice and which consequently will support your efforts to be a mindful eater. The fast I want to recommend is a "media fast." A "media fast" is a break from media—TV, radio, newspapers, magazines, the internet, maybe even your cell phone (unless you use it only to make calls). Taking a day off from all media creates the mental space for mindfulness to fill.

Shortly after the presidential election of 2016, many of my clinical psychotherapy clients became obsessed with current events. They would spend hours online or watching TV to learn what was happening and then spend hours on social media engaging in dialogue about the news. I had to "prescribe" media fasts on a daily basis to help these people find balance. You may not be a news junkie but I bet you do spend a lot of time online, watching TV, reading newspapers, etc. For one day I want you to stop and see what happens. How do you spend your time? Are you more relaxed or agitated? Is it hard for you to let go of your gadgets for even a day? Or maybe you welcome the peace and quiet. Maybe you find yourself able to meditate more deeply and longer. Maybe your taste buds are more awakened and maybe you get out of the house more! Try it for a day. If you like it, have a media fast weekly. Create the mental space for mindfulness to settle, a media fast is one way to do that.

Today: **Eat all your meals and snacks mindfully, meditate for thirty minutes and move mindfully for ten minutes.**

Today's Journal Question: **Do a media fast and describe your experience.**

AUGUST 26:

THE FOOD BALANCE BEAM

When you truly follow your Inner Wisdom, you may find that some of your food choices seem odd or unusual. You may go through periods where you find yourself eating a lot of one thing, over and over again. And, then suddenly, you are guided to something else. Sometimes the foods you are guided to are "healthy" foods. Foods you would expect to be part of a balanced diet. Other times the foods may be of the "unhealthy" variety, ones in the past you would forbid yourself from eating. Here's the beauty of mindful eating and following your Inner Wisdom—your body will not steer you wrong. There may be something inside the "unhealthy" food that your body needs to function. Who knows? Your body knows! It may be that some of your meals or snacks include foods that you previously ate mindlessly. That's okay. If you listen to your Inner Wisdom, follow its guidance and make mindful choices, over time you will eat a balanced diet. Like I said, your body won't steer you wrong.

***Today*: Eat all your meals and snacks mindfully, meditate for thirty minutes and move mindfully for ten minutes.**

***Today's Journal Question:* What are your thoughts about the idea that "your body won't steer you wrong"?**

AUGUST 27:

DOES LONELINESS MAKE IT HARD TO EAT MINDFULLY?

In my book, *The Best Diet Begins in Your Mind: Eliminate the Eight Emotional Obstacles to Permanent Weight Loss*, I assert that loneliness is one of the eight emotions that people eat over the most. When it comes to mindful eating, loneliness may be a factor too, but not only because it could lead to mindless emotional eating. Loneliness can make it hard for some people to eat mindfully, especially when they are at home. Let me explain. One of the ways to build up mindful eating skills is to eat at a table without distractions. That means no TV, radio, iPhone, iPad, etc. For people who live alone this can be tough. For many, the silence that comes with turning off all distractions can be downright painful. Sitting alone at a table with only a plate full of food in front of them hurts. Those who feel this way tell me that eating like that is too upsetting. It is a reminder of their lack of a relationship or lack of a family. Having the TV or computer on keeps them company and eases that pain. I understand that and am sympathetic.

Here's a remedy for this situation. Mindfully choose to eat your food in front of the TV, for example, and pay attention to what you are doing. Sitting across from the television set is not an excuse to eat without awareness. It is possible to savor bites while still keep tracking of who is getting a rose on *The Bachelor*. You can tune into your hunger and fullness signals even if there is car chase on *NCIS* or a fight on *Keeping Up with the Kardashians*. If you chose to eat with distractions do so with full awareness of your food. Put your food on a plate instead of eating out of a carton. Use real utensils, not plastic ones. Choose to not eat mindlessly, and instead, choose to enjoy every morsel you consume. This approach may not end your loneliness, but it will help you along your mindful eating journey.

***Today:* Eat all your meals and snacks mindfully, meditate for thirty minutes and move mindfully for ten minutes.**

***Today's Journal Question:* How does loneliness affect your eating habits?**

AUGUST 28:
YOU'RE EATING . . . WHY?

It's check-in time! How are you doing distinguishing physical and emotional hunger? Are you still eating for reasons other physical hunger? If you are, are you doing so mindfully or does mindlessness still rear its head? Please remember that mindful eating is not "perfect" eating. Mindful eating is eating with full awareness of what you are doing. If you are eating for reasons that have nothing to do with physical hunger and know exactly what you are doing and why you are doing it, you are still eating mindfully! Think about the past three days and identify how often you ate in response to physical cues and when you ate for other reasons. Other reasons might include emotional eating, being in the presence of tempting food, being offered something and not wanting to hurt the offeror's feelings or just good old-fashioned mindless eating. You are not bad if you eat when you are not physically hungry. It's just that you will manage your weight better when you stick with your Inner Wisdom.

***Today:* Eat all your meals and snacks mindfully, meditate for thirty min-**

utes and move mindfully for ten minutes.

***Today's Journal Question:* How are you doing distinguishing physical hunger from other reasons why you might want to eat?**

AUGUST 29:

SAVED BY THE BELL

If cravings overwhelm you or you found that they interfere with any diet you may tried in the past or are disrupting your efforts to eat mindfully now, take heart, you are not alone. Cravings are real experiences that can be either physical or emotional in nature. Fortunately, whatever the reason, cravings can be handled with mindfulness. The important thing to know about cravings is that they will usually go away on their own within twenty minutes, if you don't give into them. To manage cravings mindfully, try the following:

1. Recognize if you are physically hungry. If you are hungry, decide what you are hungry for and eat. If what you are hungry for is what you are craving, enjoy a portion of it mindfully.
2. If you are not physically hungry, assess if you are emotionally hungry. If you are, address your emotional need.
3. If you are not in the mood to do either of the above suggestions, simply set a timer for twenty minutes and ride the craving out. Distract yourself with some activity that does not involve food and when the bell goes off you will most likely be craving free!

If you want to learn more about how to handle cravings, I have a one-hour audio program called *7 Way to Beat Cravings* that you might find helpful. It is available through the store at TAMEYourAppetite.com/shop.

***Today:* Eat all your meals and snacks mindfully, meditate for thirty minutes and move mindfully for ten minutes.**

***Today's Journal Question:* How do cravings affect you and what are you willing to do about them?**

AUGUST 30:

NATURAL HIGH

I have a friend who loves the water. If she is not at home or working, she is in or on the water. Whether it's swimming laps, floating on rafts, sailing the high seas or splashing in water aerobics, she worships the water. I asked her once why she spends so much time in the water and she answered with a glint in her eyes, "It's my natural high. Who needs substances when you can float in water?" I looked at my friend who is healthy and slim and nodded. She was right. She had found a way to relieve her stress and cope with her life without relying on excess food or drink. Good for her! Good for you, because if she can do it so can you. So, can I. As I thought about it, I realized that walking is for me what swimming is for her. I love to walk. I walk when I am stressed. I walk when I need to think. I walk when I need a new idea. I walk when I travel. Walking is my go-to activity when I need a "natural high." Do you have a go-to activity? Do you play piano, surf, knit, paint, write, sing, draw, color? Could you? Finding an activity that you can reach for when you need a break is a wonderful way to avoid mindless and emotional eating.

***Today:* Eat all your meals and snacks mindfully, meditate for thirty minutes and move mindfully for ten minutes.**

***Today's Journal Question:* What activity could be your go-to activity to give you a natural high when you need relief from life's pressures?**

AUGUST 31:

REVIEW—WHAT IT MEANS TO BE MINDFUL

For some, mindfulness is a lifestyle. It is a way of being in the world that informs all their activities. When we are mindful, we are truly present in the moment. We experience the here and now, rather than the future or the past. When we come from a mindful place, we are better able to gain insight about who we are, what we are doing and how we are feeling. We are able to garner more understanding of those around us. We find it easier to forgive and accept. We can offer ourselves and others greater compassion and kindness. We feel more joy and peace. I hope that by now you, too, are experiencing some of these benefits of mindfulness.

***Today:* Eat all your meals and snacks mindfully, meditate for thirty minutes and move mindfully for ten minutes.**

***Today's Journal Question:* How is mindfulness operating in your life now?**

SEPTEMBER

SEPTEMBER 1:
STRESS EATING

If you are a parent, it may be the first day of school. If you are a business owner, you may be thinking about your quarterly tax bill. Whatever today holds for you, you may be feeling stressed. Stress is a common experience for most people. There are two different kinds of stress—acute and chronic. Acute stress refers to stress that comes on strong but goes away when the cause of the stress goes away. Chronic means that the stress lingers. Chronic stress can be harmful for your body. Stress can further hurt you if you use food to cope with it. If food is your go-to stress-buster, how about turning to meditation instead? How about using mindfulness to manage your stress? By using meditation and being more mindful in stressful situations you can be with your stress without having to react to it.

Here's how: Each day identify one *stressful event* as it happens. Pause, close your eyes and note the thoughts, the emotions, and sensations that occur. Then notice if any of those perceptions create an urge to do something such as: move, look away, raise your voice, or eat. Notice the urge. Feel the urge. Take a few deep breaths and then decide on how you want to respond to the stressful event. Take another full breath and open your eyes. Now, do the response you decided upon, and if it is to eat, eat. Only now you will be eating mindfully.

***Today:* Eat all your meals and snacks mindfully, meditate for thirty minutes and move mindfully for fifteen minutes.**

***Today's Journal Question:* How do you usually deal with stress?**

SEPTEMBER 2:
BODY ACCEPTANCE

Are you at war with your body? Do you wish your body looked a certain way? There may be some things you can change about your body but there are others you can't. One of things you can't change is your body type.

There are three basic body types: Ectomorph, Mesomorph, and Endomorph. Ectomorphs typically have long thin limbs, slight shoulders and narrow waists. As women they tend to be flat-chested and have delicate frames. Think Kate Moss. Mesomorphs have bigger bones, larger muscle and what we might call a "naturally athletic body." Think Serena Williams. Endomorphs have soft solid bodies. They are typically shorter with thick arms and strong legs. Think of Oprah Winfrey. As hard as she may try, Oprah will never have the same body as Kate and Kate will never look like Serena.

Which type are you and which type are you pursing? I fall into the same camp as Oprah. At five feet, three and a half inches tall and coming from hardy German and Polish stock, I will never be Kate either. So, I don't try. Sure, I wish I were five foot seven with legs to the sky, but I'm not. Never will be. Trying to obtain such a goal is pointless and yet so many of us fall into this trap. We purse lofty ideals that are unrealistic. These pursuits undermine our self-esteem and can lead to eating disorders and other maladies. Stop right now and accept your body type. Embrace what is good about you.

For me, I have very strong legs. These legs have skied the Alps, crossed the finish line of three marathons and walked the Great Wall of China. Thank you, legs. My thick arms have carried babies, injured dogs and grocery bags. Thank you, arms. I have my mother's body and am proud to come from a long line of strong powerful women. Thank you, mom. Mindfulness is about acceptance. About accepting what is. I accept my endomorphic body. I appreciate it for its wonders and work to make it the best version it can be. What about you? Can you accept your body and work towards its best version too?

***Today:* Eat all your meals and snacks mindfully, meditate for thirty minutes and move mindfully for 15 minutes.**

***Today's Journal Question:* How do you feel about your body and its type?**

SEPTEMBER 3:
YOU ARE NOT YOUR GENES

It is funny to me that I am writing this bit of wisdom to you on this day—my mother's birthday. It was not intentional, yet apropos. I want to address the role genetics have in our weight. Genetics, the biological traits we inherit from our ancestors, play a role in our health and well-being, but they are not our fate. You may have a predisposition for heart disease, for example, but that does not mean you will have an unhealthy heart. Your genes are not your destiny. The exciting field of epigenetics tells us genes can be turned on and off. Meaning that if there is predisposition for a particular trait you can activate it by your lifestyle and other factors and, similarly, you can shut it off.

This means that even if your parents are overweight, you can achieve a healthy weight. All it takes is a bit more mindfulness. You may not have a choice as to how tall you are or what color eyes you have, those genes are set in stone, but you have a choice as to how healthy or fit you are by the mindful choices you make. So, the next time you think you are doomed to have your father's potbelly, think again. Please don't use your genes as an excuse for not eating and living mindfully.

Today: **Eat all your meals and snacks mindfully, meditate for thirty minutes and move mindfully for fifteen minutes.**

Today's Journal Question: **How have you blamed your genes for your current weight and eating issues?**

SEPTEMBER 4:
MINDFULNESS TO THE RESCUE

As I got up from today's morning meditation, my left foot and lower leg cramped in a way I have never experienced before. The pain was excruciating. My leg was contorted, and I almost blacked out. I could not put any weight on it and I started to panic. All I wanted was for the pain to go away. Then mindfulness kicked and I remember what I had learned about using mindfulness for pain relief. Instead of trying to avoid the pain or force it to go away I turned my attention to it. I took several deep breaths, "breathed into the pain," and repeated the word "relax" to myself. Within moments the pain abated. I moved my foot slightly and the cramping began again. I repeated my breathing sequence and the pain receded. This happened four or five times before the pain went away for good.

Then I went on the hunt for Outer Guidance and Googled muscle cramps. I learned that dehydration and potassium deficiency are two causes for such pain. So, I drank a glass of water and ate a banana with my breakfast. As I ate the banana, I was mindful of how it was helping my body heal from muscle cramps. I was pain free the rest of the day. Mindfulness for pain relief is well-researched. If you would like to learn more, read *You Are Not Your Pain* by Vidyamala Burch and Danny Penman. It's one of the books I read as I began my mindfulness studies.

***Today:* Eat all your meals and snacks mindfully, meditate for thirty minutes and move mindfully for fifteen minutes.**

***Today's Journal Question:* What pain do you experience that might benefit from a mindfulness-based approach?**

SEPTEMBER 5:

SODA JERK

Are you a slave to your afternoon Big Gulp? Do you use soft drinks to fill you up or prevent you from overeating? Many people do. Soft drinks, or any sugary drink, lead to excess calories without satisfaction, satiety, nourishment or fullness. This can lead to more eating because your body is still hungry. You may temporarily trick your body into thinking it's full, but your body is smarter than that and in short order it will signal you to eat again. Sweetness triggers cravings, which demand that we eat or drink more. Also, sweetness damages our palate. We become so accustomed to overly sweet food products that we can no longer taste the natural sweetness of a ripe peach or slice of watermelon. Diet drinks are no better. They may trick the taste buds but not the brain and also increase our desire for sweets. Plus, there is some evidence that the artificial ingredients in some diet beverages can cause or exacerbate depression. Nobody wants that! The next time you find yourself reaching for a sweet drink, pause, take a moment to check in with yourself to determine what it is you really want. I doubt you truly want a Big Gulp.

***Today:* Eat all your meals and snacks mindfully, meditate for thirty minutes and move mindfully for fifteen minutes.**

***Today's Journal Question:* What affect do sugary drinks have on hunger, taste, satiety and fullness for you?**

SEPTEMBER 6:

WHAT DO YOU TAKE FOR GRANTED?

Occasionally at this time of year, I catch what I call a "summer cold." It's just like a winter cold, only it's warm outside. While I have this cold, I am miserable. I power through the day only to collapse into bed at night. I feel sorry for myself, sorry for those around me who have to endure my self-pity and I await the day I feel better. When that day comes, I feel so well it's like a miracle. It's only after having a cold that I appreciate the overall good health that I enjoy. Before the cold, I took my health for granted. Recognizing this helped me see how much I take for granted in general in my life.

As I embraced mindfulness, not just regarding my eating habits, but for everything, I became more aware of how fortunate I really am. There are so many things I take for granted—I can see, hear, walk, run, and breathe. I have a home, a car, a career, family and friends. I could go on, but I think you get the message. Being mindful means being aware and being aware allows us to see all the good in our lives. Let me ask you, how's your health today?

***Today:* Eat all your meals and snacks mindfully, meditate for thirty minutes and move mindfully for fifteen minutes.**

***Today's Journal Question:* What do you take for granted?**

SEPTEMBER 7:
HOW YOUR DAY AFFECTS YOUR WEIGHT

Think about a typical day in your life. Think about the people you talk to, the words you read, the music you listen to, the ads you see, the television shows you watch. Think about everything you see, hear, feel, smell and touch in any given day. All this "sensory input" we "ingest" affects us and, unless we are paying attention, unless we are being mindful, we may not even notice. The media, display ads, conversations with co-workers, tabloid headlines, news alerts, etc., seep into our consciousness and affect us deep down. If what we are taking in is negative, frightening, or devaluing, we feel bad and may not know why. Feeling bad in this way may lead us to eat to feel better. If we are eating to feel better, we are emotionally eating, and, as you know, emotional eating can lead to weight gain or slow down weight loss. It is important to be mindful of what you read, watch and hear. If watching the news disturbs you, turn it off. If looking at supermodels in fashion magazines makes you feel bad about yourself, don't look. Pay close attention to what you put into your mind as well as your body. By learning to mindfully "consume" sensory input, you can help yourself reduce unnecessary stress and negatively which can have a positive influence on your health and well-being.

***Today:* Eat all your meals and snacks mindfully, meditate for thirty min-**

utes and move mindfully for fifteen minutes.

***Today's Journal Question:* How does what you are exposed to each day affect your weight?**

SEPTEMBER 8:

ARE YOU ASLEEP AT THE WHEEL?

Have you ever walked into a room and forgot why you went in? Or have you driven past your exit on the highway without realizing it? The other day I drove my car to a friend's house in my neighborhood. Even though she lives walking distance from my home, I drove my car because I needed to run some errands before seeing her. After our visit, car keys in hand, I walked straight home. It wasn't until I got into my house that I remembered that my car was parked near her house. So, I turned myself around, walked back to her street, got into my car and drove back home. What do these examples have in common? They are all illustrations of "being on autopilot."

In other words, in those moments, we were mindless. It is time to wake up from autopilot. It is time to be more fully present in our lives. When we are on autopilot, we miss things. When we forget, we are out of touch with life. Sometimes our autopilot can be set to "numb." Numbness may protect us from pain, but we need to experience and release our pain to be whole. The next time, you walk into a room and forget why, or drive past your exit or leave your car at a friend's house, pause, take a breath, bring your attention back to the present moment and then continue with what you were doing.

***Today:* Eat all your meals and snacks mindfully, meditate for thirty minutes and move mindfully for fifteen minutes.**

***Today's Journal Question:* What are you doing on autopilot?**

SEPTEMBER 9:

DON'T SHOUT; BE CURIOUS

Have you ever overeaten and then blasted yourself for doing so? Shouting comments inside your head like, "How could you do that? Why did you eat all of it? I thought you were trying to be mindful . . ." You get the idea. Yelling at yourself for what you ate is unlikely to get you to eat less next time, but mindfulness could. Exploring your overeating with an attitude of curiosity can go a long way to ending such behavior. The next time you eat more than you want to, or foods you wished you hadn't, ask these kinds of questions in place of the reprimand, "What was I thinking when I made that choice? How was I feeling when I did what I did? How does my body feel as a result of what I ate? How did it feel before I ate it and during?"

Examining your thoughts, feelings and bodily sensations is the mindful way of investigating your eating habits. Your answers will help you interrupt future eating by creating a mindful pause that will allow you to make a different choice or not. You may still choose to eat in excess or eat foods you normally wouldn't. Either way is okay when you are being mindful. Be curious about your behavior. Inquire about your thoughts, feelings and sensations. Pry into your mindlessness and see what you uncover. In time, your inquisitive stance will lead to changes in your eating habits with very little additional effort.

***Today:* Eat all your meals and snacks mindfully, meditate for thirty minutes and move mindfully for fifteen minutes.**

***Today's Journal Question:* What does your mindlessness tell you about yourself?**

SEPTEMBER 10:

GOING BANANAS FOR BANANAS

This morning, after I came home from my morning walk, I felt hungry. I checked in with myself and decided I wanted a banana. In the past, before I became a mindful eater, I would have grabbed the banana, unpeeled it quickly and then eaten it in four or five bites as I rushed around to get ready for work. Not today! Today, I ate my banana mindfully. Today I placed the yellow-freckled banana on my placemat. I sat down, took a few breaths, and then slowly peeled the banana, one strand at a time, listening to the sound of the peel as it rolled down the side of the banana. Have you ever listened to the sound of a banana peel? I never had, until today. Then I smelled the banana. Funny, it didn't smell as I expected. It wasn't as "fruity" as I thought it would. I took a moment to reflect on the banana smell and realized that all my life I smelled artificial banana, the kind put into banana muffin mixes, banana taffy or candy. That smell was sickly sweet.

This smell was subtle, like the tropical climate from which it came.

Then, I bite into my banana and felt the soft center melt in my mouth. I took another bite and looked at the remaining part of the banana. I gently tore a piece off and admired its color and little speckles in its center. In all my years, I never admired a banana and there is much to admire—its color, its texture, not to mention the journey it took to get to me! When I finished the banana, I sat for another moment feeling grateful that I took the time to savor this banana. I had a smile on my face for the rest of the day.

Today: **Eat all your meals and snacks mindfully, meditate for thirty minutes and move mindfully for fifteen minutes.**

Today's Journal Question: **Eat a banana or other fruit today and journal about the experience.**

SEPTEMBER 11:
SPREADING PEACE MINDFULLY

September 11 is a tragic day in American history. Life changed across the globe as a result of terrorist attacks. Now we acknowledge this day by calling it Patriot Day. In honor of this day, I want to share with you how we might use meditation to bring peace to our fractured world. In 1986, December 31st was declared World Peace Meditation Day, also known as World Healing Day and the International Hour for Peace. On that day, and every December 31st since then, millions of people from around the world focus their minds on peace, loving kindness and forgiveness for an hour all at the same time.

This simultaneous meditation is believed to direct quantum energy in such a way as to create peace. It is said that meditating on peace can create peace. Dr. Jon Kabat-Zinn talks about the relationship between meditation and peace in his book titled, *Wherever You Go, There You Are*. He asserts that we can change the world by changing ourselves, specifically by focusing our attention on love and kindness we become a new "nucleus of love and kindness" which benefits the world. On this day of remembering, add some loving kindness into your meditation. Focus your attention on the prospect of lasting peace.

Today: **Eat all your meals and snacks mindfully, meditate for thirty minutes and move mindfully for fifteen minutes.**

Today's Journal Question: **How does focusing your attention on love, kind-**

ness and peace feel to you?

SEPTEMBER 12:

LET GO OF THE ROPE

When I was a little girl and went to summer camp, a popular game was tug-of-war. Tug-of-war is played with a long thick rope and two teams of campers. The rope is laid across an imaginary line and each team pulls their side of the rope until the other team is dragged across the line. If one side drops the rope, the game is over. You can't pull where there is no resistance. Little did I know then, that was my first lesson in the foundations of mindfulness. In the practice of mindfulness, we learn about acceptance. We learn about letting go and being unattached to outcomes. When you stop pulling, when you stop resisting, the battle is over. If you have been playing tug-of-war with your weight, let go of the rope. Accept where you are and take steps to improve. Let go of the struggle by allowing your weight to come off in its own time. By continuing to cultivate your mindful eating and meditation practice you will get across your finish line without pressure or strain.

***Today:* Eat all your meals and snacks mindfully, meditate for thirty minutes and move mindfully for fifteen minutes.**

***Today's Journal Question:* What "rope" can you let go of today?**

SEPTEMBER 13:

THE MIRACLE OF THE FAX MACHINE

This morning I needed to fax some documents to a company on the East Coast so that they would be waiting for my associate when she arrived at work. Given that the East Coast is three hours ahead of me, I had to go up before dawn to do this little task. In the dawn's early light and with sleep in my eyes, I went to my fax machine to take care of business. I slid the papers into the machine, punched in the phone number and pressed start. And then the miracle happened. The contents of my papers were transmitted to her fax machine in New York. I don't know if it was because I was half-asleep but I felt as if I were witnessing a miracle.

How was it possible that the information would travel in seconds across thousands of miles and an exact duplicate of what I sent would arrive on her a desk? I know—technology. Technology is itself a miracle. For the few minutes it took to send the fax I was in awe of what was happening. I was totally present for the experience. I listened to the beeping my machine made as it connected to hers. I watched as my pages slipped through the machine and the information whooshed its way across the cosmos. I paused as my machine punctuated its success with a strong tone. Until l that moment I took my old sweet fax machine for granted. In that moment I witnessed it marvelousness and the marvelousness of the universe. In that moment I was totally present. In that moment I was mindful.

***Today:* Eat all your meals and snacks mindfully, meditate for thirty minutes and move mindfully for fifteen minutes.**

***Today's Journal Question:* What everyday occurrence do you take for granted that when you think about it is a miracle you've ignored?**

SEPTEMBER 14:
SAVOR THE GOOD

As a mindful eater you are most likely savoring your food more than ever before. Tastes are lingering longer on your tongue. Aromas are inhaled more deeply. What we do with our food we can do with our life. We can savor more than freshly baked brownies or a good cup of tea. We can savor life. Our lives are filled with wonderful moments, but we don't notice them. Precious instances flicker quickly past us because our mind is somewhere else. If we stopped periodically to assess where we are, what we are feeling, and what is happening around us, our lives become richer. If we lingered a bit around that great parking spot we got before we rush into the store, or if we enjoy the music playing in the elevator as we head to appointment, or if we say thank you to a stranger who held the door for us, our lives would take on more meaning. These are ordinary moments which we typically ignore. What if you stopped ignoring them? What if you literally stopped and smelled the roses? The more present we are in our lives, the fuller we feel. And, when we are full, we don't need to eat to fill ourselves up. Today, pick a good moment and savor it. Afterwards, see how the rest of your day goes.

***Today:* Eat all your meals and snacks mindfully, meditate for thirty minutes and move mindfully for fifteen minutes.**

***Today's Journal Question:* How could savoring the good moments of your**

life help with your weight loss goals?

SEPTEMBER 15:
OUTER GUIDANCE—TO GO OR NOT GO ORGANIC

Many people ask me whether they should "go organic" or not. While I am not a nutritionist, I have done quite a bit of reading on the benefits of organic foods vs. non-organic foods. Here's what I have learned. You can use this information to guide you to make the most mindful choices for yourself. The primary reason to buy organic is to avoid the pesticides that are used to grow much of our food supply. There is science to suggest that organic foods are more nutritious for us and that are bodies are better able to utilize the nutrition within them. Some people say that organic foods taste better. One concern I hear a lot is that organic foods cost more. If cost is a factor for you, you may not want (or need) to eat all your foods organic, but you might want to do so with some of your fruits and vegetables. Each year the Environmental Working Group (EWG) puts out a list they call "The Dirty Dozen." These are the fruits and vegetables the EWG describe as having the highest concentration of pesticides and should be eaten in an organic state only. The most recent "Dirty Dozen" list I found includes these fruits and vegetables:

1. Strawberries
2. Spinach
3. Nectarines
4. Apples
5. Grapes
6. Peaches
7. Cherries
8. Pears
9. Tomatoes
10. Celery
11. Potatoes
12. Sweet Bell Peppers

If you want to eat more organic foods, this list may be a good place to start. Whichever way you choose, remain mindful and your body will guide you to the right choices for you.

***Today:* Eat all your meals and snacks mindfully, meditate for thirty minutes and move mindfully for fifteen minutes.**

Today's Journal Question: **What are your thoughts about organic vs. non-organic foods?**

SEPTEMBER 16:

WHAT COULD YOU ACCOMPLISH IF YOUR HEALTH WERE 100%?

My father used to say, "If you don't have your health, you don't have anything!" He was so right, especially after he got sick with dementia and his life went from full and consequential to empty and sad. So, I ask you, how is your health? Are you plagued with aches and pains? Do you complain of fatigue or a foggy brain? Are you struggling with a more serious condition like diabetes or cancer? Research supports the idea that mindfulness can positively affect one's health. It has been shown that mindfulness can improve such health-related behaviors as much as not smoking, getting exercise and using seatbelts. Furthermore, mindfulness can lower blood pressure, reduce depression and help deal with chronic pain. If you are still hesitant to fully embrace mindfulness, ask yourself to what could you do if your health were 100%? If that doesn't motivate you, I don't know what will!

Today: **Eat all your meals and snacks mindfully, meditate for thirty minutes and move mindfully for fifteen minutes.**

Today's Journal Question: **Answer the question, "What could you accomplish if your health were 100%?"**

SEPTEMBER 17:

NOURISH YOUR HAPPINESS

We eat to nourish our bodies. We can also do things to nourish our happiness. Happiness is actually an attitude. It is rarely truly linked to shiny objects or extreme wealth. In fact, *The World Happiness Report* (yes, there really is one) ranks countries on six factors that affect well-being: income, freedom, trust, life expectancy, social support and generosity. In 2018, Finland came in first. The United States, by the way, came in 18th. If you would like to nourish your happiness, use gratitude. This moment, before you do anything else, make a list of all the things you could be grateful for right now. All of them. Make the list long. Not sure what to write down? There are the usual things—your home, your family, your job, and your car. Then, there's your health and steady paycheck.

After you are done with the usual go-to gratitude items, think outside the box. How about being grateful for your teeth? A mouthful of teeth gives us a pleasant smile, makes eating food easier. There are people who don't have any teeth. If you do, be grateful. You can be grateful for your hands, your feet, and your eyes. How about adding freedom, independence, peace or fresh water, clean air and plenty of food to your list? Need more, use the six factors from the report above to inspire you. When you are done, notice if your mood or attitude shifted. Save your list for those days when you are feeling low. Read it over and you may feel a lightness come over you. That, my friend, is happiness.

Today: **Eat all your meals and snacks mindfully, meditate for thirty minutes and move mindfully for fifteen minutes.**

Today's Journal Question: **How will you nourish your happiness with gratitude today?**

SEPTEMBER 18:
ON THE SIDE OF THE ROAD

The other day I was stuck in traffic on LA's notorious 405 freeway. There was a multi-car accident ahead of me and my side of the freeway was at a dead stop. The opposite side however was moving briskly. I watched as cars soared out of sight and noticed that I watched some cars more than others. A sexy sports car held my attention longer than a white sedan. And I could easily let the mini-vans rush by but I strained my neck keeping the convertibles in sight. As I observed myself watch the southbound lanes cars whiz by, I was struck by the similarities between those cars and thoughts that whiz across my mind. Standing on the side of a road watching cars go by is a great metaphor for sitting on our meditation cushions watching our thoughts go by.

If you are still struggling with thoughts taking over your meditations, imagine them as cars passing by. If you are actually sitting by the side of a road and a car passes by, you don't get in, do you? No, you would just watch as it moved thorough your field of vision and then return your attention back to the road. In meditation you can do the same thing. When thoughts show up, don't "get in." Let them pass through your mind's field of vision and then return your attention to your breath. Using this metaphor helps you not attach to thoughts as you meditate. You can also practice not getting attached to your thoughts using the freeway metaphor at any time, not just when you are meditating. Give it a try.

Today: **Eat all your meals and snacks mindfully, meditate for thirty minutes and move mindfully for fifteen minutes.**

Today's Journal Question: **What thoughts can you let pass through your mind without "getting in" today?**

SEPTEMBER 19:
THE COOKING CHANNEL

A fun part of mindful eating is mindful cooking. Taking the time to shop for and prepare a meal can be a delight. There are millions of people who can't get enough of the cooking channels. Are you one of them? As I previously told you, in the nail salon I go to, the TV is almost always on the cooking channel. It doesn't matter what day or time I show up, there is someone cooking something on the screen. In the past, these shows would just be noise to be in the background of an already noisy salon. But as I was incorporating more mindfulness into my food and eating habits, I started to watch them. I paid attention to how carefully the chefs were weighing and measuring their ingredients. I listened as they described variations in spices and seasonings.

I relished in the joy on their faces as a dish came out just right. These chefs, whether they knew it or not, were engaging in mindful cooking. They were present and attentive to what they were doing. They were not multi-tasking, trying to make a soufflé while riding a unicycle. No, they just put all their attention on the soufflé. We can learn a lot from these cooking channel chefs, from how to make the perfect bouillabaisse to how to shop for zucchini. Next time you are channel surging, settle on the cooking channel and watch mindful cooking in action.

Today: **Eat all your meals and snacks mindfully, meditate for thirty minutes and move mindfully for fifteen minutes.**

Today's Journal Question: **How might mindfully cooking your meal enhance your eating experience?**

SEPTEMBER 20:

IT'S JUST ANOTHER DAY . . .

There's a song that's been humming in my head all day, ever since I heard it on the radio this morning. It's Paul McCartney's song "Another Day." It's a touching song whose chorus goes, "It's just another day. . ." If you don't know the song, search for it. If you know song, I bet you're humming it now too. I bring the song up because its chorus provides a message which we can apply to mindful eating. To truly master mindful eating and have it become what we do, we must be consistent with our efforts. Where you may fall off is with special occasions. Mindfully enjoying a piece of cake on your birthday or a fancy dinner out on your anniversary is lovely. The problem becomes when we use a special occasion as an opportunity for overeating or when these events become springboards to days, weeks or months of mindless eating. For the mindful eater, weekends, holidays, vacations, birthdays, anniversaries are "just another day."

You can certainly celebrate your special occasion and remain mindful. In fact, it has been my experience that when you are mindful, your special occasion becomes even more special because it becomes about much more than the food. In the past, a celebration may have been all about the food, but now as a mindful eater you are more aware of everything else that is happening around you and your day becomes fuller and richer as a result. If you have a special occasion coming up, think about how you could choose to be mindful and still enjoy the food associated with the event without overeating.

***Today:* Eat all your meals and snacks mindfully, meditate for thirty minutes and move mindfully for fifteen minutes.**

***Today's Journal Question:* How have you handled special occasions in the past and what might you do differently now?**

SEPTEMBER 21:

CHILDREN—THE ORIGINAL MINDFUL EATERS

When I was a grad student, we studied developmental psychology, which is psychology over the lifespan. One of the most interesting lectures for me was the lecture about children and eating. Studies showed that when left on their own, children will, over time, eat the right amounts and kinds of food they need. Children are tuned into their bodies. Given enough choices and enough time they will naturally eat in a balanced way. Problems arise when adults interfere and insist on certain foods, amounts and meal time. Furthermore, as children grow, food becomes a source of emotional support and entertainment so what was once an intuitive process is now lost among the challenges of adult life. The good news in all this is that deep down inside we are all still childlike mindful eaters. Given enough choices and enough time we, too, will eat in a balanced way. The mindful eating process you are adopting is reminding you how.

***Today:* Eat all your meals and snacks mindfully, meditate for thirty minutes and move mindfully for fifteen minutes.**

***Today's Journal Question:* Watch a small child eat and describe what you notice about their relationship to food.**

SEPTEMBER 22:

MINDFUL EMOTIONAL EATING

We have been looking at mindful meditation and mindful eating as a way to reduce or eliminate emotional eating. If your excess weight is related to emotional eating, cutting down on emotional eating will help shed some pounds. But if you find that you cannot stop emotional eating, that's fine. Many people do. The truth is food is medicine. It can work to change your mood which is why it is hard for some people to stop emotional eating. In my clinical practice, I would tell my clients that if they need to use food as a coping mechanism, they can, but to do so mindfully. Apply as many of the mindful eating skills you have been learning as possible. For example, sit at a table with a beautiful place setting. Put your food on a lovely plate. Take a few breaths. Get centered and then savor the food as you eat it. Avoid stuffing it down or eating quickly. Give yourself permission to eat emotionally if that is what you need to do, just know that is what you are doing.

***Today:* Eat all your meals and snacks mindfully, meditate for thirty minutes and move mindfully for fifteen minutes.**

***Today's Journal Question:* If you are still emotionally eating, how can eating mindfully in those moments help you?**

SEPTEMBER 23:

CREATING RIPPLES

Probably the most charitable person in our lifetime was Mother Teresa. Known for her devotion to others, she exemplified selflessness. I heard a quote from her once. She said, "I alone cannot change the world, but I can cast a stone across the waters to create many ripples." She was describing interconnectedness. Mindful eating can help us understand how we are all interconnected. The pear you had for a snack today came to you because of this interconnectedness. Someone planted the seed that grew the tree. Someone picked the pear from the tree. Someone transported the pear to the market you got it from. Someone placed it in a bin for sale. Someone took your money to pay for it. And, of course, Mother Nature played her role too. Without water, sun or soil, that pear would not exist. In the busy, frenetic, mindless world we live in, it is easy to forget that what we are all connected and that what we do affects others. Even a simple smile can have positive ripple effects.

Let's say you pass a stranger on the street and as you see her you smile. Just a polite, we are both on the same street at the same time, smile. Your smile may have just brightened what might have been a difficult day. Now she is in a slightly better mood when she gets to work and as a result is kinder to a customer with a complaint. This customer feels heard and satisfied that her problem got resolved and she goes home and has the patience to help her son with his homework. He gets an A on his next exam and his self-esteem soars. All this happened because you smiled—the ripple effect. Today, keep in mind the notion that we are all connected and that even a small seemingly inconsequential act can have a big effect. Send out a ripple.

***Today:* Eat all your meals and snacks mindfully, meditate for thirty minutes and move mindfully for fifteen minutes.**

***Today's Journal Question:* How can you create ripples today?**

SEPTEMBER 24:

A DAY IN THE LIFE OF YOU

Back in the 1990s, the *A Day in the Life of . . .* books were popular. These books displayed a city's life through captivating photographs. I recently came across one that I have about New York City and seeing that book made me muse what a day in my life would look like if a photographer followed me around. Then, I thought of you and wondered, what is going on in your daily life? And, more importantly for our purposes, how mindful are you throughout your day? How much of your day are you aware of and how much is autopilot? I must admit that as much as I am studying and practicing mindfulness, I am on autopilot a lot. From my morning routine getting ready for the day, to driving wherever I need to go, to checking my cellphone whenever I have a break. Today, however, I did less of that. Today, because I was reminded of the importance of being present in my life, I paid more attention. I did things slower. I questioned myself before I picked up my phone to assess whether I really needed to look for text messages again. Because I made myself more conscious, I had a lovelier day. I felt calmer, less pressured and, dare I say, happier. What would happen if you spent your day being more mindful? What would your *A Day in the Life of* book contain?

***Today:* Eat all your meals and snacks mindfully, meditate for thirty minutes and move mindfully for fifteen minutes.**

***Today's Journal Question:* As best you can, try to spend today being more aware of what you are doing and what's happening around you and then reflect on your experience.**

SEPTEMBER 25:
APPLE SEASON

Autumn is apple-picking season for us in the northern hemisphere. Now is the time to taste dozens of varieties of the crispest, most delicious apples Mother Nature offers. Now is also the time to do an apple meditation. If you have the chance to go apple picking, I suggest you do. Spending time in an apple orchard can expose you the interconnectedness of our food and our lives in a way that shopping in the market can't. Whether you pick your own apple from a tree or pick one up at your local farmer's market, get ahold of an apple and prepare to be delighted.

- Take your apple to a special spot where you can eat it without being disturbed.
- Pick up the apple and hold it between your hands. Feel its weight.
- Look at it. Notice its colors and textures. Feel its texture against your skin.
- Bring it to your nose and notice its scent.
- Place it to your lips and take a bite. Hold the bite in your mouth,

but don't chew. Feel it. Roll it over your tongue. Notice the bite mark your teeth left behind.

- Now, chew the apple and notice its flavor. Chew slowly and intentionally noticing how the apple's taste and consistency change.
- When you are ready, swallow and feel the apple slide down your throat.
- Place your hand on your stomach and imagine the bite of apple settling there.
- Take another bite and savor the apple's taste and texture.
- Continue to eat the apple slowly and deliberately.
- If you start to feel full, you can stop eating the apple. When you stop sit for a moment reflecting on the joy eating the apple brought you.
- If you are not full, finish the apple. Rejoice in the experience of being fully present for this delightful piece of fruit.

***Today:* Eat all your meals and snacks mindfully, meditate for thirty minutes and move mindfully for fifteen minutes.**

***Today's Journal Question:* Describe in your journal the experience of eating an apple mindfully.**

SEPTEMBER 26:

IS THAT YOUR STOMACH RUMBLING OR YOUR HEART?

How are you doing recognizing the difference between physical and emotional hunger? Have you uncovered any triggers that start you eating or continuing to eat when you don't really need to? Being able to separate these two kinds of hunger, and respond to each in a mindful manner, is the crux of ending unnecessary eating and achieving the weight that is right for you. I bring this topic up again now because this is probably the most important, and maybe most difficult, skill to master.

One way to know the difference between these two hungers is this—when you are physically hungry you will gladly eat celery or a cucumber or even a kumquat. But when you are emotionally hungry you won't. It is more likely that when you are emotionally hungry you want something sweet and gooey or hot and spicy. So, the next time you are feeling as if you "want to eat something" ask yourself if a carrot will do. If the answer is no, you are most likely looking to quash an emotion and the more mindful approach would be to figure out what it is. Keep working on this skill, I am confident that you will get good at it.

Today: **Eat all your meals and snacks mindfully, meditate for thirty minutes and move mindfully for fifteen minutes.**

Today's Journal Question: **What gets in the way for your recognizing the difference between physical and emotional hunger?**

SEPTEMBER 27:
STILL WAITING FOR WEIGHT LOSS

Today we will revisit the issue of weight loss. In the beginning of this yearlong journey, I talked to you about using the scale as a tool for feedback about how your mindful efforts were going. Have you been weighing yourself? If so, how frequently? Has the frequency of your weighing been serving you? During these past nine months our focus has been on changing your relationship to food. Each day we have been looking at different aspects of life and different elements of mindful eating and seeing how they merge. While weight loss is an ultimate goal, it is not THE ultimate goal.

Yes, if you practice mindful eating, your body will find its way to the weight that is right for you and you will also receive the gift of peace with food which for me, and for many others, is the ultimate gift. I once heard it said that if you focus on mindfulness, you will lose your weight but if you focus on your weight, you will lose your mind! Funny but in some ways true. If you do weigh yourself, try your best be neutral about the number. Use it as feedback and nothing else. With patience and persistence, you will arrive at your "right size" body.

Today: **Eat all your meals and snacks mindfully, meditate for thirty minutes and move mindfully for fifteen minutes.**

Today's Journal Question: **How are you using the scale during this journey?**

SEPTEMBER 28:

YOU DON'T NEED WILLPOWER, YOU NEED ATTENTION

Back in May I brought up the issue of willpower and the work of Dr. Roy Baumeister. I want to revisit this topic because so many people are still "white knuckling" their way through the weight-loss process. Are you? Let's take a look at Dr. Baumeister's famous study using cookies and radishes. In this study, the research participants were placed in a room that smelled of freshly baked cookies. Two platters were put in front of them. One had the cookies. The other the radishes. One group was told to snack on the cookies. The other group was only allowed the radishes. After their snacks, both groups were given a puzzle to complete. The radish group quit after only a few minutes, while the cookie group mustered on. Dr. Baumeister concluded that the radish group could not finish the puzzle because they had exerted too much willpower resisting the warm cookies leaving them drained and depleted. Can you see how that happens? Do you understand that relying on willpower will not really help you? Rather than trying to gather your inner strength to avoid that warm plate of cookies, use your Inner Wisdom instead. Are you doing that or are you still trying to power through? Be honest.

***Today:* Eat all your meals and snacks mindfully, meditate for thirty minutes and move mindfully for fifteen minutes.**

***Today's Journal Question:* How much are you still relying on willpower to change your eating habits?**

SEPTEMBER 29:

SPACES IN BETWEEN

There is a famous quote attributed to Holocaust survivor and author of *Man's Search for Meaning*, Viktor Frankl, which is, "Between stimulus and response there is a space. In that space is our power to choose our response. In our response lies our growth and our freedom." I don't know if Dr. Frankl knew anything about mindful meditation when he made this statement, but it describes what happens when we develop a meditation practice. We create the space for us to choose our response. Mindfulness and mindful meditation allow us to act intentionally rather than react impulsively. The more mindful our choices, the better they serve us.

This is the key to managing our emotions, engaging in healthy behavior, and improving our interpersonal relationships. This is the key to not eating when you feel emotional and to cope with the emotions directly. As you continue in your meditation practice, look for those spaces where you can deliberately choose for yourself what would serve you best in that instance. Practice interrupting reactive, impulsive actions and replacing them with thoughtful deliberate ones. Practice noticing these spaces in between and watch your behavior change.

Today: **Eat all your meals and snacks mindfully, meditate for thirty minutes and move mindfully for fifteen minutes.**

Today's Journal Question: Describe how being able to create space between a thought, an emotion and/or an action can serve you.

SEPTEMBER 30:

OUTER GUIDANCE—SUGAR AND FLOUR

There is a lot of controversy about whether we should or should not eat sugar and flour. Some experts claim that those ingredients are the worst substances for us, while other say they are just fine. So, how do you know if sugar and flour are right for you? Use a combination of Outer Guidance and Inner Wisdom. Using the guidelines for recognizing good versus junk science I introduced to you on July 20, do your research. Then, using your Inner Wisdom as your guide, experiment on yourself. How do you feel after eating sugar? Hyper, sleepy, fine? What about flour? Does flour agree with you? If you are interested, check out different types of flours—wheat, rice, garbanzo bean (yes, that's real!). Remember, with mindful eating there are no good or bad foods, there are only foods that are good or bad for you.

Today: **Eat all your meals and snacks mindfully, meditate for thirty minutes and move mindfully for fifteen minutes.**

Today's Journal Question: **How do you feel about sugar and flour?**

OCTOBER

OCTOBER 1:

HOW COMMITTED ARE YOU TO YOUR MEDITATION PRACTICE?

By now you may be sick of my saying that meditation is the foundation of mindful eating. But it is. Meditation is what makes mindful eating different than intuitive eating and other weight management techniques. By teaching the mind how to focus on the present and by calming the body down, meditation allows for a more peaceful relationship with food and your body. If meditation is so important, and if research supports that the more you meditate the more successful you will be with mindful eating I ask, how is your meditation practice going? Are you practicing regularly? Have you slacked off?

With mindful meditation all you have to do is begin again. If you have been following along with my recommendations for what to do each day, you are up to thirty minutes a day. If not, where did you fall off? Go back to that point and begin again. If that feels too hard, go back to the very beginning and begin again with one minute, then three, then five, then ten and so on. If it helps, get a new cushion to sit on or download a new meditation app. Enroll in some classes or sign up for a retreat. Do whatever you need to do to begin again. Keep beginning again and your practice will take root.

Today: **Eat all your meals and snacks mindfully, meditate for thirty minutes and move mindfully for twenty minutes.**

Today's Journal Question: **How have your feelings towards meditation changed since you first began?**

OCTOBER 2:

THE BRAINS HAVE IT

Our brains are miraculous organs. They control everything from our breath to our thoughts and whatever is in between. Dr. Sandra Aamodt, author of *Why Diets Make Us Fat*, explains that our brains regulate our weight using several different systems and that dieting puts those brain systems in conflict with each other. She further declares that diets lead to mindless eating in part because dieting teaches us to become more responsive to external cues and less responsive to internal cues. Mindful eating, she says, gets us out of that trap by focusing our attention inward. She further asserts that mindful eating puts those systems back into alignment. Her conclusion is that mindful eating is a better long-term strategy for weight management than dieting. Dr. Aamodt's work is further support that you are taking the right course of action by learning mindful eating. Keep it up. You are three-quarters of the way through your first year of mindful eating. Good job!

***Today:* Eat all your meals and snacks mindfully, meditate for thirty minutes and move mindfully for twenty minutes.**

***Today's Journal Question:* How does knowing that mindful eating helps to realign your brain after years of dieting assist you in this journey?**

OCTOBER 3:

WHEN THE FOOD STOPPED SINGING MY NAME

For most of my adult life (before mindful eating that is), my world revolved around food—what would I eat, what I would not eat, what I ate, you know the drill. Food would be on my mind most of the time, like an annoying hum or earworm that I couldn't shut off. Then, one day, I noticed it had shut off. My mind was no longer preoccupied with food, in any way. The food stopped singing. Now, the only time I think about food is when I start to feel physically hungry. I am no longer planning what I will eat for lunch at breakfast, or what I will eat tomorrow, today. My mind now is free to think of other things. My mind is at peace with food. I often talk about mindful eating leading to feeling at peace with food, and this is one way it happens. No more preoccupation. No more judgment or worry. I think about food when it is time to eat. The battle is won. The war with food is over.

***Today:* Eat all your meals and snacks mindfully, meditate for thirty minutes and move mindfully for twenty minutes.**

***Today's Journal Question:* Has food stopped singing to you? If yes, how does that feel? If no, what could you do to help it stop?**

OCTOBER 4:

OPEN 24 HOURS A DAY

Frank Sinatra famously sang that New York is a city that never sleeps. Well, I have news for Frank—we now live in a world that never sleeps. It doesn't matter what time it is; you will find a store open, a website to browse, a TV show to binge-watch. Long gone are the days of blue laws which required stores to be closed on Sundays. I am all for advancement, and technology is my friend, but this 24/7 life we live has its drawbacks. Being "on" all the time creates expectations and stress. It is no longer acceptable to take an hour to return a phone call, email or text. We want our response now! Advertisers know this better than most and they thrive on it. Ads create a sense of urgency and in our up-all-the-time culture, we can act on those urges easily.

Giving into these impulses can result in excess shopping, excess drinking and excess eating. How do we find peace in this fast-paced setting? You guessed it. With mindfulness. Mindfulness creates the pause we all need in our lives to avoid rash, impulsive actions. Mindfulness allows us to stop, think, consider and then make a choice. So, whether it is deciding to buy shoes at 4am or bite into a frozen Snickers bar for dinner, remember to be mindful and you will make the right choice for you.

***Today:* Eat all your meals and snacks mindfully, meditate for thirty minutes and move mindfully for twenty minutes.**

***Today's Journal Question:* How can being mindful help you to make better choices in our 24/7 world?**

OCTOBER 5:

THE ANGRY EATING RESPONSE

Eating when we are angry is a common occurrence. How often have you ripped open a bag of chips and shoved a handful in your mouth as you cursed the heavens over the latest atrocity to befall you? I am being a bit dramatic here but I suspect you know what I am talking about. When we are frustrated and cannot give voice to what is hurting us, we may turn to food to squelch the feelings. Fortunately, there is something else you can turn to when you are angry—meditation. Mindful meditation has been shown to be an excellent tool for not only dealing with anger as it arises but research also shows that a regular meditation practice can make you slow to anger in the first place. With meditation you can identify when you are angry, you can monitor your bodily sensations that accompany it, and most important you can be present with it without having to act on it.

Through meditation, you learn to observe your anger without judgment. It becomes just another thought or feeling that you neither cling to nor run away from. By creating this space around anger, you can make a mindful decision on how to respond to the situation that provoked it. You stop reacting automatically and instead respond purposefully. Now that is what I call peace of mind.

***Today:* Eat all your meals and snacks mindfully, meditate for thirty minutes and move mindfully for twenty minutes.**

***Today's Journal Question:* What role does anger play in your eating and weight issues?**

OCTOBER 6:
MINDFUL GIVING

When I was a little kid, my mom would ask my sister and me to go through our toys to choose items we no longer wanted so we could give them to children who were not as fortunate as we were. These donations were my entry into the world of giving. Later as an adolescent I would put together neighbor shows and "carnivals" in our driveway. I would charge a small fee to attend and all the money would go to charity. At Halloween, I would trick-or-treat with a UNICEF contribution can in one hand and my candy-filled pumpkin in the other. I learned early on the value of giving. In the Buddhist tradition, in which mindfulness finds its roots, generosity is one of its basic customs. Being generous with your money, your time or your talent can be a mindful practice.

When you intentionally give of yourself to others you are being mindful. The next time you are in a funk over your eating, your weight, or how your body looks, make a decision to give. Find an object you possess and give it to someone else who might appreciate receiving it. Or offer to do a chore or errand for someone who might not have the time or resources to do it for herself. Put an extra dollar in the next tip jar you come across or give someone a genuine compliment. Practicing mindful giving feeds us in ways that food never can. Mindful giving serves both you and the recipient. Allow yourself to feel the joy that giving elicits. It is sweeter than sugar.

***Today:* Eat all your meals and snacks mindfully, meditate for thirty min-**

utes and move mindfully for twenty minutes.

***Today's Journal Question:* What can you give today?**

OCTOBER 7:
EAT A MEAL IN SILENCE

In our open-all-night world it is very rare to experience total silence. Even in the dead of night you can hear air conditioning units humming, refrigerators turning on and off, cellphones buzzing. And when we eat there is usually a lot of hubbub going on around us pulling our attention away from the plate in front of us. The first time I was at a silent retreat, the silence was disconcerting. I had never been around so much silence. But once I got used to it, I appreciated it. One thing I noticed was a heightening of my other senses. My vision seemed clearer and my hearing more acute. What was especially noticeable was how good the food tasted when I ate in silence. Because my attention was not straying off course, I could focus more on the food and its flavors. Try it for yourself. When possible, eat a meal or snack in total silence. No music. No TV. No conversation. Just quiet. Notice if the experience is different than usual. Notice if you eat more or less food than you might otherwise eat. Notice if the flavors stay strong longer. Eating a meal in silence is a wonderful event. Once you try it you may never go back to noise.

***Today:* Eat all your meals and snacks mindfully, meditate for thirty minutes and move mindfully for twenty minutes.**

***Today's Journal Question:* Eat a meal or snack in silence today and reflect upon your experience.**

OCTOBER 8:
OUTER GUIDANCE—DIABETES AND MINDFUL EATING

Today I got a call from a client who told me that he has been diagnosed with diabetes. He said his doctor is sending him to Lifestyle classes that will include nutritional counseling. He asked how this news will affect his mindful eating efforts. I explained that this is a perfect example of using Outer Guidance to inform one's mindful choices. For example, let's say he learns that eating food high in sugar is not in his best interest, he can use that information to help him make decisions about what to eat. He and I did a little exercise. I asked him to imagine that he was hungry as he was checking in with himself deciding what to eat. I told him to imagine he had two choices that would be equally satisfying—pecan pie or trail mix. Because his Outer Guidance has taught him that high-sugar items are not good for him, he could choose the trail mix. Of course, he is free to choose the pecan pie but now he does so knowing that his Outer Guidance is recommending against it. He chuckled and said that the trail mix would be fine, it's one of his favorite snacks. With that said, I suspect he will be just fine.

Today: **Eat all your meals and snacks mindfully, meditate for thirty minutes and move mindfully for twenty minutes.**

Today's Journal Question: **If you learn that you have a medical condition that restricts your dietary choices, how will you use this Outer Guidance to help you make mindful choices?**

OCTOBER 9:
USING FOOD TO CONNECT WITH OTHERS—THE MINDFUL POTLUCK

There is no denying that food plays an important role in our society. Put aside the issues of diet and weight loss and think about how food is a universal connector. Food rituals bond cultures. Family meals strengthen relationships. Neighborhood barbecues bring community together. Today I would like you to use food as a way to connect with others. I would like you to organize a potluck. For your potluck, invite four to six people to your home and ask each to bring a favorite dish. If it helps, you can create categories and assign a guest to each category. For example, if your pot luck is a dinner, one guest could bring an appetizer, another an entrée, a third a side dish, a fourth a dessert, fifth a beverage, and so on.

At the potluck, ask each guest to describe the dish they brought and why they chose that particular one. Spend a few moments appreciating each of the guests and their contributions before the meal starts. When eating, savor the food, acknowledging the different tastes and textures represented. If your guests are also mindful eaters you could add in a mini-meditation and eat part of the meal in silence. The purpose of this potluck is for you to feel how food can bring people together, what effect that might have on your eating and how eating with others can be seen as a sacred or spiritual event.

***Today:* Eat all your meals and snacks mindfully, meditate for thirty minutes and move mindfully for twenty minutes.**

***Today's Journal Question:* Organize a potluck and reflect on the event in your journal.**

OCTOBER 10:
WHO NEEDS COUPONS WHEN YOU HAVE MINDFUL EATING?

A funny thing happened on the way to the market. I discovered that I didn't need so many bags. What am I talking about? Here, in Southern California, we need to bring our own reusable bags when we grocery shop. Someone somewhere made it so that stores were prohibited from providing single-use plastic carryout bags to customers. So, being the good SoCal gal I am, I loaded up on canvas tote bags, always keeping at least six in the trunk of my car. Whenever I went to the market, I would take my bags with me, and, in the old days, I would fill up most them. Then something started to change. I was bringing too many bags. Each grocery trip yielded fewer items so fewer bags were used. I noticed something else—my weekly grocery bill was slowly decreasing. Suddenly, the light went on. Being a mindful eater, paying close attention to my hunger, fullness and satiation signals, has resulted in my eating less food, naturally, and without forced effort. Hence, the few items, fewer reusable bags, and lower bills. This happened slowly over time without any deliberate action on my part, other than practicing my mindful eating skills. Who knew mindful eating could save money?

***Today:* Eat all your meals and snacks mindfully, meditate for thirty minutes and move mindfully for twenty minutes.**

***Today's Journal Question:* How has your grocery bill changed since becoming a mindful eater?**

OCTOBER 11:
YOUR HEALTHY BRAIN

Dr. Dan Siegel, world-renowned neuroscientist, created *The Healthy Mind Platter* which describes seven categories of activity for optimal brain and body well-being. They are Focus Time, Play Time, Connecting Time, Physical Time, Time In, Down Time, and Sleep Time. Each of these categories can be a valuable tool in mindful living. When we engage in Focus Time we are concentrating on a particular task. In Play Time we allow ourselves to be creative and have fun. With Connecting Time, we interact with people or the environment around us. During Physical Time we move our bodies. Time In is reflective time. Down Time is relaxation time and Sleep Time is, of course, when we restore ourselves through sleep. When practiced mindfully, each of these categories can improve our lives, enhance our well-being and support our efforts to be a mindful eater. How many of these categories do you engage in regularly? What can you add that would improve your well-being?

Today: **Eat all your meals and snacks mindfully, meditate for thirty minutes and move mindfully for twenty minutes.**

Today's Journal Question: **How could implementing The Health Mind Platter improve your life?**

OCTOBER 12:
UNTIL THE COWS COME HOME

As a child growing up on Long Island, I had the luxury of a stay-at-home mom for most of my formative years. That meant I was met each day with milk and cookies after school. Milk was a staple in our house as it was for so many others. In the 1990s, the "Got milk?" ad campaign drew a lot of attention for the dairy industry and for a while created a surge in milk consumption. Now, in the 21st century, some people are examining the wisdom of drinking milk. Whether to include milk or other dairy products into your diet is a question that necessitates both Inner Wisdom and Outer Guidance to answer. There are those who suggest that it is unnatural to drink cow's milk since we are not cows. There are others who avoid milk products because of their perspective on how the dairy industry treats their animals.

For some, dairy products cause severe gastrointestinal pain because of lactose, the sugar found in milk, so they omit it. Then, there are those who prefer a vegan or vegetarian diet and avoid all animal products. If you are questioning whether to include dairy among your food choices, do some homework. If you agree that humans shouldn't drink cow's milk, take milk off your list of mindful options. If dairy presents an ethical dilemma for you, by all means make your smoothie with almond milk instead of yogurt. And if you are one of those who is lactose-intolerant, then you may choose to avoid dairy products because your body is shouting No! to you in no uncertain terms. As with all foods, it is your choice whether to choose to eat them or not based on your own Inner Wisdom and Outer Guidance. There is no right or wrong choice. The only choice that counts is your unique mindful choice.

***Today:* Eat all your meals and snacks mindfully, meditate for thirty minutes and move mindfully for twenty minutes.**

***Today's Journal Question:* If you are questioning whether to include dairy among your mindful food choices, what sources of Outer Guidance can you research?**

OCTOBER 13:
DOES YOUR ENVIRONMENT SUPPORT YOU?

Dr. Kelly D. Brownell, a renowned scientist from Yale University, studies weight and food-related matters. Some of Dr. Brownell's research focuses on the relationship between environment and obesity. His findings are important. Whether we talk about our society's environment or your unique environment at home and work, we must to be mindful of the effects from our surroundings. For example, keeping a bag of chips in plain sight is more likely to lead to mindless eating, than storing it in the cupboard. Similarly, displaying a large bowl of fresh peaches might remind you to choose fruit instead of fries the next time you are hungry.

Our environment provides cues that lead us to eat. From commercials on TV to donut trays in the staff lounge to drive-thru fast-food chains on almost every corner, we can be triggered to eat food we are not hungry for. While it is not possible to avoid all environmental cues, you can be strategic about your environment. For instance, carrying healthy snacks in your bag or briefcase can prevent you from grabbing that donut. Choosing restaurants with healthy choices when dining with friends can make being mindful easier. And keeping a copy of this book where you can see it can be a reminder of your efforts to be a mindful eater.

***Today:* Eat all your meals and snacks mindfully, meditate for thirty minutes and move mindfully for twenty minutes.**

***Today's Journal Question:* How does your environment support or hinder your weight loss efforts?**

OCTOBER 14:

GETTING YOUR ZZZS

Did you know that sleep affects weight? If you don't get the right amount of sleep for your body, you may gain weight. There are several reasons for this occurrence. First, lack of sleep increases fatigue which leads to less movement and less movement can notch up the scale. Second, that same fatigue can cause excess eating because we reach for food for energy to get us through the day. Third, with less sleep we are up more hours during the day which can also lead to more eating because we have more opportunities to grab something. And fourth, lack of sleep decreases appetite control hormones which results in an increase in our hunger signals, which lead to more eating, especially high carb/high calorie foods. If you have trouble with sleep I have good news for you, mindfulness can help.

Remember the Body Scan meditation I taught you back in March? Practice it again. This meditation is especially helpful for insomnia because it releases tension in your body and helps you relax. You can even practice it in bed to drift you off to sleep. If relaxing your body isn't enough to get your baby blues down for the count because it is your ever-busy mind keeping you awake, practice the mindfulness technique of watching your thoughts rather than engaging them.

To do that, simply notice them, label them as thinking, questioning, worrying (whatever label fits) and then watch them drift away. It is clinging to thoughts and then imaging an entire scenario around them that keeps you up. Let them go. They will be there in the morning if you still need them. If none of these suggestions help, you may want to try Mindfulness-Based Insomnia Therapy (MBIT). It is a cognitive-behavioral approach based in mindfulness. I have my version of an MBIT program in the store at TAMEYourAppetite.com. It is an audio-visual program called *Sound Mind, Sound Sleep*.

***Today:* Eat all your meals and snacks mindfully, meditate for thirty minutes and move mindfully for twenty minutes.**

***Today's Journal Question:* How do your sleeping habits affect your weight and your eating activities?**

OCTOBER 15:
RESILIENCY

Resiliency is the ability to recover from crisis or other turmoil quickly and effectively. A resilient person has the ability to cope well with hardship and come through difficult situations whole. Resilient people are not born that way; they become that by learning different ways of thinking and behaving. An excellent way to become more resilient is through meditation. Pausing and watching the mind, as we do in mindful meditation, teaches us to resist getting trapped in the minutiae of our lives and fosters the ability to respond in constructive ways. Through your meditation practice, you learn to handle unpleasant emotions and pestering thoughts without becoming burdened by them. So, if you still need another reason to develop a meditation practice, here it is.

***Today:* Eat all your meals and snacks mindfully, meditate for thirty minutes and move mindfully for twenty minutes.**

***Today's Journal Question:* During one of your meditation sessions, repeat this phrase to yourself and then describe how you feel afterwards: "Regardless of what is happening, I can deal with it."**

OCTOBER 16:
HOW'S YOUR HANDWRITING?

My maternal grandmother had the most exquisite handwriting. Each stroke looked like a calligrapher had crafted it. I loved receiving cards and letters from her. They were especially glamorous because she wrote in German. I, on the other hand, have a terrible handwriting. It wasn't always bad. It got bad in law school (remember, I started there!) because I had to write copious notes during each class lecture, and over time I became a scrawler. Years later I had the opportunity to interview a handwriting analyst and I asked her what I could do to improve my handwriting. Expecting her to tell me to practice calligraphy or get a keyboard, she simple replied "slow down." She continued, "The only reason for poor penmanship is speed." Busted! She was right.

When I slow down, I have nice handwriting. Not as beautiful as my grandmother's but certainly legible. I was reminded of her comments earlier today when I tried to read some notes I had written to include in this book for you and I couldn't figure out what I had written. I was guilty of mindless writing! It got me thinking how mindlessness infiltrates all aspects of our lives and that if we simply slowed down, we would fare much better. Today I vow to write slower. I also vow to drive slower and pay more attention when I walk. What do you do so quickly it borders on mindless and how can you slow down?

***Today:* Eat all your meals and snacks mindfully, meditate for thirty minutes and move mindfully for twenty minutes.**

***Today's Journal Question:* Use your journal today to practice your handwriting and see what difference slowing down makes.**

OCTOBER 17:
SWEET SWEET POTATO

It was a relatively cool day here in Southern California. Not the blistering cold in the Midwest, but cold enough that I wanted some "comfort food." When I considered what I wanted to eat for dinner, an image of a sweet potato popped into my head. I have been mindfully eating long enough by now to know that my Inner Wisdom was speaking to me. I went to my cupboard and saw that I had two sweet potatoes left. Perfect! I grabbed the potatoes and then considered what else I might want along with the potatoes to complete my meal. Just then, the image of the sweet potato popped into my head again. Could it be that all my body wanted was the sweet potatoes?

Historically, meaning before mindful eating, I would naturally have prepared what would be considered a "balanced meal"—a sweet potato, some green vegetables and a piece of chicken or fish. But not today. Today my Inner Wisdom was guiding me just to the sweet potatoes. So, I obeyed. I took the potatoes to the sink and gently scrubbed them one at a time feeling the brush in my hand and the water trickle down my fingers. Then I wrapped each potato in some foil and admired the shiny objects I had created. I turned my oven on to 450 degrees, placed the potatoes on the rack and walked away. I busied myself with other tasks until the smell of cooking sweet potatoes caught my attention.

Suddenly I felt warm and cozy. I went to my kitchen to retrieve my dinner. I placed the still wrapped potatoes on a plate and took it to my place setting. I sat down. Carefully, I unwrapped each sweet delicacy and admired my handiwork. Slowly, I ate the potatoes, savoring each delicious bite. When I was done, I felt full, satisfied, and content. Who knew that eating only one food for a meal could work so well? That is the beauty of mindful eating.

***Today:* Eat all your meals and snacks mindfully, meditate for thirty minutes and move mindfully for twenty minutes.**

***Today's Journal Question:* What is your reaction to eating only one food as an entire meal?**

OCTOBER 18:
USING YOUR BODY TO STAY PRESENT

It is easy to be mindless. Your goal in this journey can't be to be mindful all the time. That's impossible. We are humans after all and we have minds that never turn off. Instead, a goal I would recommend is to be mindful most of the time. What can you do if you are caught up in mindlessness? Use your body to get grounded in the present. Wherever you are and whatever you are doing, stop and notice your body. Sit or lie down and direct your attention to your body and feel it rest upon the carpet, tile, or bed. Let your body sink into the surface to remind yourself that you are here, now, in this moment. Take a breath and assure yourself that this moment nothing else matters but you and your body. Spend a minute or two anchoring yourself in the present by feeling your body. When you are done, go on with your day. Repeat this as often as necessary to keep you in the moment.

***Today:* Eat all your meals and snacks mindfully, meditate for thirty minutes and move mindfully for twenty minutes.**

***Today's Journal Question:* The next time you notice you are being mindless, bring yourself back to the present moment by focusing on your body and reflect on how that helped you in your journal.**

OCTOBER 19:
EVEN GOODWILL DESERVES BETTER THAN THAT

You are ten months into your mindful eating experience and now I think it is time to make some changes. Years ago, when I was doing work as a psychology and law expert on television, I hired an image consultant to help me get "camera-ready." She came to my house to sort through my clothes and accessories to see what I could wear for my appearances. Curious and a bit nervous, I welcomed her into my master bedroom to rummage through my closets and drawers. Over the course of several hours, she inspected every blouse, dress, t-shirt, suit, you name it, that I owned and strategically sorted all the items into three piles. The first pile was the "you can keep this" pile. The second pile was the "this goes to Goodwill," and the third pile was called the "even Goodwill deserves better than that" pile. The third pile was the largest by far.

Stunned, I watched as she tossed all the clothes and accessories from piles two and three into large garbage bags. What was left was a modest assortment of clothes, shoes and handbags that fit me perfectly, looked nice on me and I felt good in. Getting rid of all the items that were stained, torn, outdated or the wrong size was a leap of faith but one that I was glad I took. Today, I'd like to suggest that you too create an "even Goodwill deserves better than this pile" and rid yourself of all the items in your wardrobe that no longer serve you. We did a clutter exercise back in July, but just in case you didn't tackle your clothing at that time, or you have accumulated more in the intervening months, today would be a good day to mindfully assess your wardrobe and then lovingly save, donate or toss your stash.

***Today:* Eat all your meals and snacks mindfully, meditate for thirty minutes and move mindfully for twenty minutes.**

***Today's Journal Question:* What can you save, donate, or toss today?**

OCTOBER 20:
7 TYPES OF HUNGER

Dr. Jan Chozen Bays, in her book *Mindful Eating: A Guide to Rediscovering a Healthy and Joyful Relationship with Food*, describes seven different types of hunger: eye, nose, mouth, mind, heart, stomach, and cellular. According to Dr. Bays, each of these affects why we want to eat. We want to eat when we see (eye), smell (nose) or taste (mouth) something appealing. We also eat when our thoughts (mind) and emotions (heart) tell us to (mind). And we eat when we feel physically hungry (stomach, cellular) or the body requires something specific. Mindful eating is eating from stomach and cellular hungry. The other hungers trigger reactive or mindless eating. At this stage of your mindful eating journey, you are most likely pretty tuned into these different kinds of hunger but there is value in reviewing how you are doing. For today, notice what type of hunger prompts you to eat. Are you still reacting to external cues or are you more tuned into your body's Inner Wisdom?

***Today:* Eat all your meals and snacks mindfully, meditate for thirty min-**

utes and move mindfully for twenty minutes.

***Today's Journal Question:* What role do Dr. Bays' seven hungers play in your current eating patterns?**

OCTOBER 21:
TEA CEREMONY

One of the nicest moments I ever shared with my mother was when we were in Japan and participated in a Japanese tea ceremony. A Japanese tea ceremony is one of best demonstrations of mindfulness I can think of. This tradition begins with the host sending out formal invitations to her guests followed by preparing her home for the ceremony. These preparations include cleaning the room in which the ceremony will take place. If it is summertime, it may be the garden. The host also prepares the items she will use and any food she may serve. In addition, the host prepares spiritually for the event. The guests prepare too. Both the host and the guests are advised to leave behind all their daily concerns and open their minds and their hearts to what will occur.

As the guests enter the tea room, they wash their hands, bow as a sign of respect and take their seats. Using traditional gestures and movements the host then washes the items she will be using for the tea. No unnecessary movements or talking occurs. It is a sacred moment. Everything is in harmony. She then prepares the tea in a bowl to serve to her guests. The first guest receives the tea bowl, takes a sip, wipes the rim and passes the bowl to the next guest. Each guest follows suit until all have sipped from the bowl.

When the ceremony is complete the host washes the items again and the guests acknowledge her work. The guests bow as they leave. The sanctity and serenity of such an event needs to be experienced firsthand to truly appreciate its wonder. If you ever have a chance to engage in tea ceremony, I encourage you to do so. You can create your own version by steeping a pot of tea for yourself and some friends, serving it in your most elegant cups and the drinking it silently while rejoicing in the glory of the moment.

***Today:* Eat all your meals and snacks mindfully, meditate for thirty minutes and move mindfully for twenty minutes.**

***Today's Journal Question:* Describe about how a tea ceremony such as the one I described is an embodiment of mindfulness.**

OCTOBER 22:
WISDOM FROM PEMA CHODRON

There is an American Buddhist nun named Pema Chodon who teaches at a Tibetan monastery in Nova Scotia. She also writes books. One of her books is called *Taking the Leap: Freeing Ourselves from Old Habits and Fears.* In the chapter titled "Learning to Stay," she eloquently describes ways to practice being present. She writes:

"One way to practice staying present is to pause, look out, and take three breaths. Another way is to simply sit still for a while and listen. Simply listen to the sounds in the room. For one minute, listen to the sounds in the distance. Just listen attentively. The sound isn't good or bad. It's just sound."

With the world clamoring around us, what a lovely way to be mindful. I offer this to you today as a way of deepen your mindfulness practice by reminding you of the simple ways we can "learn to stay."

***Today:* Eat all your meals and snacks mindfully, meditate for thirty minutes and move mindfully for twenty minutes.**

***Today's Journal Question:* Listen to the sounds around you, what do you hear?**

OCTOBER 23:
SHARE MINDFULNESS WITH A FRIEND

The kids these days talk about having BFFs—best friends forever. If you have a BFF, how about sharing with them the gift of mindfulness? I call it a gift because mindfulness has the potential to positively affect all aspects of our lives. What other gift can do that? You can share mindfulness in many ways. Here are some ideas: (1) Give your friend a copy of this book as an introduction to mindfulness; (2) Invite them to join you for a meditation class at a local yoga center; (3) Attend a half-day retreat together; (4) Sit them down and guide them through their first meditation session; and (5) have a heartfelt discussion of how embracing mindfulness has helped you make changes in your life.

***Today:* Eat all your meals and snacks mindfully, meditate for thirty minutes and move mindfully for twenty minutes.**

***Today's Journal Question:* With whom will you share mindfulness today?**

OCTOBER 24:

KEEP READING

Back in May I recommended that you spend a few minutes day reading something what would enhance your journey to mindfulness and mindful eating. Did you do that? If you have, I hope that what you read did indeed help you along in this process. If you did not, it is not too late to start. Once again, I would like to encourage you to devote a few minutes, or pages, a day, to "contemplative reading." If you are wondering what to read, you might enjoy books from some of the authors I mentioned earlier: Jon Kabat-Zinn, Jack Kornfield, Jean Kristeller, Andrea Lieberstein, Thich Nhat Hanh, Kristen Neff, and Sharon Salzburg.

You can also include the other authors I wrote about in some of these daily passages. If not, go to Amazon and search mindfulness and mindful eating for ideas. As I suggested earlier, you might like to assemble a few friends to form a book club and read these books together. Whichever book you choose to read, keep an open mind, a non-judgmental stance and pay attention to the words on the page. In other words, read mindfully!

***Today:* Eat all your meals and snacks mindfully, meditate for thirty minutes and move mindfully for twenty minutes.**

***Today's Journal Question:* If you have been reading about mindfulness and mindful eating, write about how what you have been reading has influenced your mindful eating journey.**

OCTOBER 25:

MINDFUL EATING AND ITS EFFECT ON THE WORLD

A beautiful outcome of mindful eating is that many of us become more aware of the effects our food choices have not only on ourselves but also on the world. When we start to pay attention, we notice how the animals we chose to eat are raised. We see the consequences our food choices have on global-warming and the rainforest. Because we are more tuned into the process of how the food we eat comes to us, we feel more a part of the worldwide community. Mindful eating also makes us more compassionate, balanced and accepting which can have a ripple effect on all of humanity. By being present, aware and in the moment, we can be more responsive to what is going on around us and act in a way that spreads peace and kindness. The simple act of mindful eating could change the world. Want to be a part of that change?

Today: **Eat all your meals and snacks mindfully, meditate for thirty minutes and move mindfully for twenty minutes.**

Today's Journal Question: **How can your mindful eating choices positively affect the world we live in?**

OCTOBER 26:

THE ROAD BEAUTIFULLY TRAVELED

I just arrived in Phoenix from Los Angeles to attend a professional conference. The hotel I was staying in was about a half-hour from the airport, so I called for a cab and headed out. After handing the driver my bags, I settled into the back seat and pulled out my phone. I was about start checking emails and text messages when something caught my eye. There, right outside my passenger window, was the tallest, most beautiful cactus I had ever seen. Catching a glimpse of that magnificent plant jolted me out of my mindless activities and into the moment. I had been in Phoenix once before and suddenly remembered how beautiful it is, how different the scenery is from LA. So, I put my phone away and turned all of my attention to the sights outside the window. From the mountains in the distance to the cacti lining the highway, I was mesmerized. By making the choice to be present for this car ride, I was able to enjoy all it had to offer. By the time I arrived at my hotel, I felt energized and excited, instead of tired and travel-weary. It's amazing what a mindful decision can do.

Today: **Eat all your meals and snacks mindfully, meditate for thirty minutes and move mindfully for twenty minutes.**

Today's Journal Question: **What do you see when you look outside the passenger window of a vehicle you are riding in?**

OCTOBER 27:

THE WONDERS OF DINING ALONE

It is the first day of the professional conference I am attending in Phoenix and since I came by myself to this event, when I went for breakfast, I dined alone. I travel solo often so I am comfortable asking for a table for one, but I know some people aren't. If you don't like to eat out alone, let me tell you about what I did so you can see how you might enjoy solo dining the mindful way. To begin with, dining alone is the best opportunity to practice mindful eating. Talk about no distractions. It is easy to take your time reading through the menu, noting the different options to choose from. If the restaurant offers a cuisine that you do not regularly eat, explore the ingredients and spices in the unusual menu items. Because I was in Phoenix, this menu had all sorts of southwest-style options—huevos rancheros, breakfast burritos, corn, and bean hash. I checked in with my Inner Wisdom for guidance on what the right choice for me might be and settled on the breakfast burrito.

After placing my order, I set my sights on the restaurant's décor—giant tapestries depicting the Arizona sun, lovely hand-crafted pottery, and Western-style candlestick holders. In a word, gorgeous. When my meal was served, I centered myself, took a few deep breaths and then admired the platter in front of me. On display were two halves of the burritos, each teeming with scrambled eggs, cheese, tomato, and corn. Draped over the burrito halves were salsa and thin slices of avocado. I lifted one of the halves, raised it to my lips, deeply inhaled its flagrant aroma, and bit in. I ate slowly, savoring each delightful bite.

When I finished the first half, I asked myself if I wanted the other. My answer was no, I was comfortably full and didn't need anymore. Truthfully, if I had been with companions, I might not have noticed that I was full and mindlessly eaten the whole thing. Instead, I got a to-go box, placed the remaining half inside and took it with me as a snack or meal for later. My entire dining experience was pleasant, peaceful and enjoyable. And, because I was eating mindfully, I was able to easily stop when I was full, consuming the right amount of food for me at that time.

***Today:* Eat all your meals and snacks mindfully, meditate for thirty minutes and move mindfully for twenty minutes.**

***Today's Journal Question:* If you don't like to dine solo, what could you do to make such an experience enjoyable?**

OCTOBER 28:
MINDFUL PREPAREDNESS

In psychology we use the term "denial" to explain a person's inability to be present with some kind of truth. It is an unwillingness to face facts. In mindfulness terms, it's being mindless. Today I am reminded of a manner in which all of us may be mindless and that is with respect to being prepared for emergencies. In Los Angeles, where I live, we need to be prepared if an earthquake strikes. That means we need to have supplies such as food, water, flashlights and batteries, ready in the event we are without power or resources. In the southeast, you need to be prepared to evacuate in the event of a hurricane. In the Midwest you need a tornado plan.

For many of us, myself included, we think about getting prepared, we may even create an emergency kit and then we forget about it. We go mindless. When we have small tremors, I am reminded about my need to be prepared and then I forget again. Today I chose to remember. This morning before doing anything else, I reviewed my "Earthquake List." This is a list I have ready which identifies what essentials I need to take from with me in the event I need to evacuate my home because of earthquake damage. I updated the insurance, medical and financial information. I made sure I knew where everything was and put the list with my passport and emergency cash in a safe place. Now I am ready. What can you do today to get prepared for a possible emergency? What potential event have you chosen to ignore or deny that needs your attention? Take time today to be mindfully prepared.

Today: **Eat all your meals and snacks mindfully, meditate for thirty minutes and move mindfully for twenty minutes.**

Today's Journal Question: **What possible emergency do you need in order to be prepared?**

OCTOBER 29:

BEGIN . . . AGAIN

As we round out October (month ten of our journey together) I want to remind you that you can always begin again. Whenever you falter, begin again. Been eating mindlessly for days, weeks, even months? Begin mindful eating again. Eat one bite of food mindfully. Haven't meditated since the spring? Sit on your cushion for one minute and begin meditation again. Not answering your journal questions? Answer today's question and begin writing again. Your only exercise is finding the remote when it falls under the couch? Take a five-minute walk and begin moving again. If you have stopped doing any healthy habits, begin it again. Simply, easily, mindfully. There is no judgment here. No contest. No failures. Only awareness, mindfulness and a willingness to begin again.

***Today:* Eat all your meals and snacks mindfully, meditate for thirty minutes and move mindfully for twenty minutes.**

***Today's Journal Question:* Reflect upon which mindful habits you may have stopped doing and how you can begin again.**

OCTOBER 30:
BUDDHA AND THE HUNGER GHOST

In the Tibetan *Book of the Dead*, there is a parable about the Hungry Ghost. This ghost has a huge stomach and a tiny neck and mouth. The challenge for the Hungry Ghost is that it can never be satisfied. It cannot eat enough to fill its enormous belly and this insatiability is extremely painful. It never gets what it desires. For the Hungry Ghost there is only yearning, craving and deprivation. In Buddhism, the Hungry Ghost is a metaphor for spiritual emptiness and addiction. In Western culture, the Hungry Ghost is often tied to Halloween and is sent away by the jack-o-lantern placed by your door.

Have you ever felt like a hungry ghost? Do you feel as if you cannot get enough? Do you have unfilled desires? To some extent, we all have needs that go unmet. Trying to get rid of these unmet needs usually backfires. Sometimes our efforts only reinforce the craving or desire. Instead, the way to tame the Hungry Ghost is through acceptance and gratitude. By accepting what is and expressing gratitude for what we do have, we can heal the Hungry Ghost within us. So, the next time you go in search of satisfying a craving, try meditating on acceptance and gratitude instead.

***Today:* Eat all your meals and snacks mindfully, meditate for thirty minutes and move mindfully for twenty minutes.**

***Today's Journal Question:* Is there a Hungry Ghost inside you? If so, what are its desires and what will you do about them?**

OCTOBER 31:
HAPPY MINDFUL HALLOWEEN

Welcome to the best or worst day of the year depending on how you feel about having candy in your home. For those of us who can't be around a Snickers bar without biting in, Halloween can present many challenges unless you approach it mindfully. Today marks the end of the tenth month of building mindful eating and living skills. This day has the potential to be your best Halloween ever. To show yourself that you can trust yourself around Halloween treats, I want you to get a few pieces of your favorite candy. Go ahead, I'll wait. Once you have your candy assembled, you will go through a mindful eating exercise that will show you that you can eat candy without losing all control.

- Begin by placing your candy on a beautiful candy dish or plate.
- Admire the candy on the plate. Pay attention to the colors of the wrappers if it's wrapped.
- Choose one piece to start with and pick it up.
- Look at it. Notice its colors and textures. If it is wrapped, unwrap it. Linger over the unwrapped candy paying attention to how it looks.
- Next, bring the candy to your nose and sniff. How does it smell?
- Touch it to your lips. Feel its texture.
- Place it in your mouth, but don't chew. Feel it. Roll it over your tongue.
- Bite into it. Notice its flavor.
- Chew it but don't swallow.
- Now swallow and feel the food slip down your throat.
- Place your hand on your stomach and imagine the bite of food settling there.
- Now look at your plate again. Choose another piece of candy and go through the steps again.
- Repeat these steps with each candy on your plate or until you feel as if you have had enough for this sitting.
- When you are finished, give yourself credit for eating the candy slowly and mindfully. Remind yourself you can eat candy this way every time you have some.

Today: **Eat all your meals and snacks mindfully, meditate for thirty minutes and move mindfully for twenty minutes.**

Today's Journal Question: **Which Halloween treats would you like to enjoy and why?**

NOVEMBER

◆◆◆

NOVEMBER 1:
IF YOU HAVE TO ASK

Probably the most challenging part of being a mindful eater is being a mindful stopper. Meaning, stopping yourself from eating more when you have gotten the fullness signal from your Inner Wisdom. I know that is hard to stop eating, especially if what you are eating is really delicious, formally forbidden or hard to come by. For many, this is the biggest stumbling block to reaching their weight-loss goals. One way I trained myself to stop eating is to notice when I was asking myself if I wanted more. I concluded that if I had to ask, I didn't! Do I want more . . . salad, crackers, popcorn, ice cream, whatever, became a signal for me that I have had enough. I knew this to be true because other times I naturally reached for more without any hesitation or deliberation. At those times, after I ate the additional portion, I felt satisfied and could easily walk away from the table. Try the "if you have to ask" approach and see if that helps you stop when your body tells you it has had enough.

***Today:* Eat all your meals and snacks mindfully, meditate for thirty minutes and move mindfully for twenty-five minutes.**

***Today's Journal Question:* Are you able to stop eating when you reach comfortable fullness? If yes, why yes? If not, why not?**

NOVEMBER 2:
COPING WITH HOLIDAY TREATS

Over these next two months, we will be looking at the holiday season and how mindfulness can help you manage all that is heading your way. This is the time when holiday-specific foods, foods which we typically do not eat at any other time of the year, show up. This makes these foods more special, more appealing and more likely to lead to mindless or emotional overeating. Today, I want to help you break the link between a holiday and its associated foods. The best way to approach these holiday delicacies is the same way you have been practicing approaching all food—with awareness. Of course, I want you to enjoy your grandma's baked ham or your sister's noodle kugel, and by now you know very well that when you eat food mindfully, paying attention to your Inner Wisdom, you will eat less and enjoy your food more. Serve yourself your favorite foods and choose to eat them slowly, without distraction, savoring each and every bite. If you are mindful in this way, you can enjoy your holiday treats and know that you will come into the New Year without the typical 5-pound weight gain which everyone else will be complaining about.

Today: **Eat all your meals and snacks mindfully, meditate for thirty minutes and move mindfully for twenty-five minutes.**

Today's Journal Question: **Write down the mindful eating steps and techniques that you will use this holiday season.**

NOVEMBER 3:
LOVING THE ONE YOU'RE WITH

The holiday season can be stressful for families and other relationships. If you want to weather a pending family feud, do a loving kindness meditation. Thinking about the person with whom you have trouble, repeat to yourself, "I wish joy and happiness for this person." Then remind yourself that you are doing the best you can and show compassion and kindness toward yourself. These simple actions can go a long way to soothe tensions, promote cooperation, and foster harmony. This loving kindness meditation is not only for the holidays. Use it any time you have difficulties with a person in your life.

Today: **Eat all your meals and snacks mindfully, meditate for thirty minutes and move mindfully for twenty-five minutes.**

Today's Journal Question: **Whom can you offer some loving kindness to today?**

NOVEMBER 4:
LEARNED HELPLESSNESS

Have you ever wondered why a gigantic 6-ton circus elephant can stay tethered to a small chain and not run off? The answer is because the elephant learned that he cannot break free of the chain. How did the elephant learn that? He learned that as a small elephant when tied to a post with a huge chain. Try as he might, the baby elephant could not break free of the chains, so over time, the elephant learned that he cannot break free from any chains. This phenomenon is known in psychology as learned helplessness. Learned helplessness does not only affect elephants. It affects us humans too. We learn that no matter what we do about a particular situation we can't make it better so we stop trying. I see many clients who demonstrate learned helplessness around their weight. They have failed so many times at managing it they feel as if they can't. If this sounds like you, don't give up! Learned helplessness is just that—learned. If it is learned it can be unlearned and mindful eating is your teacher.

Taking a mindful approach to a situation you feel you cannot change means to observe the situation with curiosity and investigation. If the adult elephant were able to do that, she would see that she is much bigger and stronger than the chain that binds her and she could set herself free. If you take a look at what is holding you back, I bet you will find that it is not bigger or stronger than you, you just think it is. Your excess weight may seem bigger and stronger than you are, but it isn't. You may feel tethered to your weight the way the elephant felt tethered to her chain, but you are not. Weight is just weight and weight comes off when the body is properly nourished, well-treated and in balance. Explore your weight loss efforts with a spirit of curiosity and open-mindedness. What do you learn? How thick is your chain? Are you sure you can't break free of it?

***Today:* Eat all your meals and snacks mindfully, meditate for thirty minutes and move mindfully for twenty-five minutes.**

***Today's Journal Question:* How have you learned to be helpless?**

NOVEMBER 5:
SHOPPING LIKE A EUROPEAN

I was very lucky. I had the good fortune to spend ten months living in beautiful Bologna, Italy. I was an undergraduate student at the time, taking classes at the Johns Hopkins University's School of Advanced International Studies, known as SAIS (remember I was a lawyer before becoming a psychologist). SAIS was a graduate school so there were no dorms for me to stay in. I, along with three classmates, shared an apartment in the center of the city. Since there was no dorm, there was no dining room. Consequently, my roommates and I had to fend for ourselves. This meant shopping for groceries. In Bologna, at least at the time I was there, there were no mega-sized supermarkets. Instead, the streets were lined with shop such as bakeries, fruit markets, butchers, and cheese stalls.

To gather groceries, we would go from shop to shop buying what we needed. There were no shopping carts or cars with roomy trunks to carry our load, so we learned to shop in small quantities more often. As a result, the food was fresher, we had less waste and our choices were more varied than they might otherwise have been. Returning to America, I went back to my American way of shopping for a week or month at a time at a mega-store. That is until I became a mindful eater.

As a mindful eater, I am more in tune with what my body wants to eat at a particular time. I am no longer creating weekly menus or following a prescribed food plan, so my food choices are more spontaneous. I tried loading up my house and fridge with lots of choices but discovered that much of that food went to waste because I was eating less. Instead, I decided to shop like a European. I now buy smaller amounts of food more often to ensure that I have the freshest versions of whatever food my body wants. Yes, that means more trips to the market, but those trips are quicker and, for me, well worth the extra effort.

Today: **Eat all your meals and snacks mindfully, meditate for thirty minutes and move mindfully for twenty-five minutes.**

Today's Journal Question: **What can you do to shop like a European?**

NOVEMBER 6:
WOULD YOU LIKE A MINT?

Do you have a sweet tooth? Do you believe that a meal without dessert is no meal at all? Very often I feel as if I want something sweet after a meal too. In the past, that probably would have a piece of cake, a bowl of ice cream or some pie. Now I respond to my "need" for something sweet after a meal differently. Now, I have some mint. After dinner mints are nothing new. Restaurants have been giving diners mint candies with their bill for decades. Hotels leave chocolate mints on pillow cases. There is something about mints that is wonderfully satisfying. My mint of choice is a half stick of Doublemint chewing gum. I few minutes of having the mint flavor in my mouth is usually enough to quench my desire for sweets. A cup of mint tea is also nice, especially if I am out to dinner and others are ordering dessert and I'm not partaking. Perhaps something minty will work for you too. Give it a try. You have nothing to lose except for maybe garlic breath.

***Today:* Eat all your meals and snacks mindfully, meditate for thirty minutes and move mindfully for twenty-five minutes.**

***Today's Journal Question:* How do you feel about mint after a meal or snack?**

NOVEMBER 7:
WHAT WILL YOU ELECT TODAY?

The Tuesday after the first Monday in November is Election Day in America. On this auspicious day, we get to cast our ballots for candidates and issues that reflect our values and goals. As a mindful eater, you too get to cast your vote in a way that reflects your values and goals each time you "elect" to eat something. Every sip, lick, taste and bite is a vote, a choice. You can choose to eat foods that align with your Inner Wisdom or you can decide to ignore that assistance. Just like the choice of whom and what you vote for is yours alone, so are your mindful and mindless choices. They are yours and just like with an election, sometimes you win and sometimes you lose. How will you execute your right to "vote" today?

***Today:* Eat all your meals and snacks mindfully, meditate for thirty minutes and move mindfully for twenty-five minutes.**

***Today's Journal Question:* How do you decide on what, when and how much to eat?**

NOVEMBER 8:
IF IT WERE A SNAKE, IT WOULD BITE YOU

In the classic television show *I Love Lucy*, there is an episode in which the character Fred Mertz, played by William Frawley, can't find his glasses, even though they are sitting atop his head. When he discovers them, he says, "If they had been a snake, they would have bitten me." I just had my very own

Fred Mertz moment. I was sitting at my computer typing away when I needed to look up a reference in a book. I pulled the book off the shelf, reached for my glasses but they were not there. I turned over papers, looked under the bookcase, tossed by purse but I couldn't find them.

Then, aggravated, I put my hand on top of my head, as if to say, "What now?" and felt the metal frames. I burst into laughter. Here I was writing messages about mindfulness when I had a clearly mindless moment. I share this with you so you know that "mindless happens." Even well into your mindfulness journey, you will be mindless. The next time it happens to you, please think of Fred and me, and burst into laughter. You are in good company.

***Today:* Eat all your meals and snacks mindfully, meditate for thirty minutes and move mindfully for twenty-five minutes.**

***Today's Journal Question:* Are you expecting that because you are a student of mindful eating and mindfulness, you will never falter and have mindless moment? Why or why not?**

NOVEMBER 9:
THE BLINDFOLDED MEDITATION

This morning I did an experiment. While sitting for my morning meditation I covered my eyes. I used an eye mask that you wear for sleep. I had one in my travel bag and wanted to see what it would be like to block out all the light that comes in through my eyelids. I know what you must be thinking, "This woman has too much time on her hands!" Maybe so, but I was still curious, so I tried it and I am so glad I did. The added darkness enhanced my meditation experience. Sometimes I get distracted by the shadows I see through my eye lids and those distractions remove me from my practice. Today that didn't happen. I did distract myself sometimes by noticing the darkness but I can report that my whole meditation experience was richer. If light pulls you out of your meditation practice, try using a mask as I did. If noise bothers you, try ear muffs or ear plugs. Remove whatever distractions get in your way and see if you enjoy your meditation more.

***Today:* Eat all your meals and snacks mindfully, meditate for thirty minutes and move mindfully for twenty-five minutes.**

***Today's Journal Question:* Meditate today with an eye mask or ear plugs and reflect on the experience in your journal.**

NOVEMBER 10:
TRAIN METAPHOR

A few years ago, Los Angeles opened its Metro rail service. For those in New York, Chicago or Boston this may not be a big deal but for commuters in LA it was a game changer. Among the changes are railroad crossings. Now, when we are driving in our cars we need to stop for trains. As I approached one of these crossings and came to a stop as the guard rails lowered, I was reminded of a meditation exercise I was taught as I was learning to meditate. It was the train metaphor. In it I was instructed to see my thoughts as train cars passing by. The idea was to let the thoughts pass without "getting on." While at the crossing, I watched as the train whizzed by reflecting on how fleeting it (and my thoughts) were. If you would like to try the train metaphor, here is a brief meditation for you to use:

> *Become comfortable in your chair and gently close your eyes. Allow your shoulders, chest, and stomach to relax. Focus your mind on the feeling of your breathing. Take two or three deeper breaths from your diaphragm, letting the air flow all the way into your stomach and then flow gently back out again.*
>
> *Now imagine that you are standing on the platform of a train station. Look around the train station, what do you see? What do you hear? Now imagine trains passing by. See them pass without your stepping on.*
>
> *Now imagine that your thoughts are like those trains racing by the station.*
>
> *Observe each thought, whatever comes to mind. No judgment. Just observation. Rather than focusing on the thought and thinking about where it will lead—which is like stepping onto the train and going wherever the train is headed stand back and observe the thought. Where did it come from? Is it positive or negative? Where is it going?*
>
> *If you engage the thought, imagine as if you have stepped onto a train and gently bring yourself back to the platform. Gently return yourself to the platform each time you notice a thought.*
>
> *Now, bring your attention back just to the breath, back to body. Gently move around and when you are ready, open your eyes.*

***Today:* Eat all your meals and snacks mindfully, meditate for thirty min-**

utes and move mindfully for twenty-five minutes.

***Today's Journal Question:* How can viewing your thoughts as passing trains help you in your meditation practice?**

NOVEMBER 11:

YOU ARE A VETERAN

Today is Veteran's Day in the United States. On this national holiday, we honor and remember those who served our country through our armed forces. Even if you have never been part of the military, you are still a veteran, and that's because a veteran is generally defined as a person who has had a lot of experience in a specific subject or discipline. You, my friend, are a veteran of many topics that are food and diet related. You are most probably a veteran dieter. You may be a veteran chef or baker. You could be a veteran tennis player, aerobics participant or yoga enthusiast. You might even be a veteran couch potato, but today, we celebrate your being a veteran mindful eater. You are almost a whole year in. That's a lot of experience. I bet, if pressed, you could give a one-hour talk on mindful eating based on everything you have learned so far. Today, as we pay tribute to those who have made America safe, please pay tribute to yourself by honoring the work you have done and the efforts you have made to master mindful eating. You worked hard, you sacrificed, and you deserve some recognition.

***Today:* Eat all your meals and snacks mindfully, meditate for thirty minutes and move mindfully for twenty-five minutes.**

***Today's Journal Question:* How can you acknowledge the efforts you have made to become a mindful eater?**

NOVEMBER 12:

MEMORY IN A CUP

Today, for some reason that I could not initially understand, I wanted some coffee-flavored ice cream. I usually don't eat coffee ice cream but today I honored my desire and got some. I served the ice cream in a pretty tea cup and sat down to eat it. I picked up a spoonful of the caramel-colored delight and placed it in my mouth. Then I slowly pulled the spoon out wiping the ice cream along my tongue. OMG! So delicious. As I savored my creamy treat, I remembered the many times my father had coffee ice cream. Coffee ice cream was his favorite flavor and he would order it whenever he had the chance. While writing this book, my father passed away from dementia. The last time I "spoke" with him it was hardly a conversation. My sister put the phone to his ear and I could hear him mumble but he was not able to respond to me. I miss my dad very much. As it turned out the coffee ice cream was like a memory in a cup. Food is like that. It can evoke memories—good and bad. This is why it is so valuable to be mindful of our food; to be connected to it so we can have these memories. Now that I think about it maybe I chose to have coffee-flavored ice cream because tomorrow would have been my father's ninety-fifth birthday and it was my way of celebrating with him. Happy birthday, Dad!

***Today:* Eat all your meals and snacks mindfully, meditate for thirty minutes and move mindfully for twenty-five minutes.**

***Today's Journal Question:* What food memories do you have?**

NOVEMBER 13:
FRIDAY THE 13TH

There is a superstition among some of us raised in Western culture that Friday the 13th is an unlucky day. The superstition may go as far back as the Middle Ages. You may be wondering why I am bringing up the idea of this day being unlucky. You may be asking what luck has to do with weight loss. Well, some people believe that one has to be lucky to be thin. That it's the luck of the gene pool lottery that determines who stays thin and who gains weight. I disagree. Back in September, I told you about epigenetics. If you remember, epigenetics is the scientific study of how our genes are turned on and off.

According to epigenetics, we may have a predisposition for some trait or condition, but we may or may not experience that trait or condition unless something turns on (or off) the corresponding gene. What you eat, where you live, who your friends are, how much you sleep and how athletic you are can cause your genes to turn on or off. To me, this is good news. Instead of being saddled by heredity, we can take action to support a healthier body and higher quality of life. In other words, we can make our own luck. So, just because mom and grandma are overweight doesn't mean you will have to be overweight too. Practicing mindful eating, mindful movement and meditating could help turn off (or prevent turning on) the genes that influence how much you will weigh.

***Today:* Eat all your meals and snacks mindfully, meditate for thirty minutes and move mindfully for twenty-five minutes.**

***Today's Journal Question:* What are your beliefs about genes, heredity, and weight?**

NOVEMBER 14:
WHEN IN DOUBT, BE GRATEFUL

Bad days happen. We all have them. The car gets a flat. The kids miss the school bus. Your boss wants that report yesterday. When you are ready to throw your hands up in the air and don't know what to do, be grateful. Gratitude has been a running theme in our journey. Gratitude works. Gratitude helps. Gratitude puts things into perspective. Once we have perspective, we are better able to come up with workable solutions. And once we have a workable solution, we are less likely to stress or emotionally eat. Having a bad day? Be grateful for what is going right. Got a headache? Be grateful for the health in the rest of your body. Hard up for cash? Be grateful for the money you do have. When you don't know what to do, how to feel or what to say, find something to be grateful for. Expressing gratitude is so simple and yet unbelievably effective. Give it a try.

***Today:* Eat all your meals and snacks mindfully, meditate for thirty minutes and move mindfully for twenty-five minutes.**

***Today's Journal Question:* How might being grateful help you avoid stress or emotional eating?**

NOVEMBER 15:
MINDFUL EATING ON AUTOPILOT

Did you read the title of today's lesson correctly? It says mindful eating on autopilot, not mindless eating. Up until now, eating on autopilot typically meant eating without awareness or eating out of habit without regard to what your Inner Wisdom might suggest. Today, I want to know if your mindful eating is on autopilot, but now, I am defining autopilot as being second nature. In other words, have you been practicing mindful eating so much that it is what you do without much forethought or effort? I hope so! Ultimately, that is the goal—for mindful eating to be how you eat from now on. If mindful eating is your go-to way of eating, if it's become a new habit, congratulations you have arrived. If it isn't, no problem. Keep on practicing and you will get there, and once you get there, you won't want to ever turn back.

***Today:* Eat all your meals and snacks mindfully, meditate for thirty minutes and move mindfully for twenty-five minutes.**

***Today's Journal Question:* Is your mindful eating on autopilot yet? If it isn't what can you do to get it there?**

NOVEMBER 16:

ONE BAD APPLE

It was late on a Friday afternoon and I felt hungry for a snack. In my mind I surveyed what would meet my body's needs at that time and settled on an apple. Sitting on my dining room table was a bowl filled with three shiny red apples. My mouth watered in anticipation of my snack. I chose one of the apples, sat down at the table and took a bite. Yuck! The apple was mushy inside. I like hard crisp apples that making a crackling sound when you bite into them. This apple was not good by my standards, so I decided not to eat it and reached into my bowl for another. With great expectations, and a bit more hunger, I bite into apple number two. Another bad apple. What is going on here? How can both apples be bad? Confused, I reached for apple number three. I studied it. It looked firm and healthy. I squeezed it a few times to see if it saw soft. It wasn't so I took a bite.

As soon as my teeth bite past the peel, I heard the sound I was waiting for—crunch! This was a delicious apple. A smile broke out on my face as I took another chomp into my sweet treat. It took three tries to find the right apple. It was worth the effort. But what if I only had two apples and they were both bad—what would my choices have been? I could have chosen not to eat either apple and tuned into my Inner Wisdom for help. Or I could have chosen to eat the bad apple knowing fully that I was making a choice that might meet my nutritional needs but might not be that satisfying. Fortunately, I didn't have to do either of those since I had the third apple. With the third apple resting comfortably in my belly and the other two disappointing apples in the trash, I went to the store to get new apples for tomorrow. I made sure to get three.

Today: **Eat all your meals and snacks mindfully, meditate for thirty minutes and move mindfully for twenty-five minutes.**

Today's Journal Question: **What foods have you eaten even though they didn't taste good and why?**

NOVEMBER 17:

MINDFUL EATING IS GOOD FOR YOUR DIGESTION

Dr. Kelly Brogan, author of *A Mind of Your Own*, recommends mindful eating for the positive influence it has on digestion. She says, on page 167, that "a quiet, settled atmosphere promotes ideal digestion. . . ." She continues, "your digestive processes will be compromised if you share your eating time with distractions such as watching TV, checking email, or getting engaged in heated discussions." Dr. Brogan is right. How many times have you gobbled down your lunch while answering emails and phoning a friend, only to be sidelined with heartburn later on? Or how many times were you so distracted that you ate much more than your body needed and had a stomachache by the end of the day? Before mindful eating, I could attest to both those scenarios. Taking the time to quiet yourself down, turning off your distractions and settling into your meal is good for body, mind and soul. And you won't need to keep Tums in every drawer or at the bottom of all of your purses anymore.

Today: **Eat all your meals and snacks mindfully, meditate for thirty minutes and move mindfully for twenty-five minutes.**

Today's Journal Question: **How does eating mindfully or mindlessly affect your digestion?**

NOVEMBER 18:

MINDLESSNESS CHECK-IN

A few days ago, we explored whether your efforts to become a mindful eater have resulted in your new eating habits being on autopilot or not. Today, we will revisit where in your life are you still mindless? In other words, where in your life are you still acting strictly out of habit when that habit may no longer serve you? For example, do you mindlessly check your iPhone every few minutes for new texts or tweets? Do you drive in a way that you miss your exit or even your driveway? Do you text and drive? How about your daily routines? Do you always wear the same suit and tie or pair of shoes simply because they are there? Do you throw all your laundry into one load and hope for the best? Do you toss your bills into a drawer, forgetting them until it's too late? We are all mindless from time to time, that's human nature, but are there things you do that, if you were paying better attention, would work out better for you? Maybe you want to pay attention to those?

***Today:* Eat all your meals and snacks mindfully, meditate for thirty minutes and move mindfully for twenty-five minutes.**

***Today's Journal Question:* Where are you still being mindless and what might you do about it?**

NOVEMBER 19:

INNER WISDOM REVISITED

After developing a consistent meditation practice, recognizing and honoring your Inner Wisdom is probably the most important mindful eating skill you can acquire. In fact, if all you do is listen to your Inner Wisdom, you could change your eating habits in a dramatic way. So, let's review. How does your Inner Wisdom talk to you? How do you know when you are hungry, thirsty, full, and satisfied? Are the signals clear? Or are they still fuzzy? Go back to the lessons about Inner Wisdom and focus your attention again on those areas that are not quite there. Remember this is a work in progress. It doesn't matter how long it takes for you to trust and obey your Inner Wisdom. All that matters is that you keep trying. You'll get it. You'll see. Once you are tuned into your Inner Wisdom regarding your food and eating habits, you might notice that your Inner Wisdom offers assistance on other matters as well. You might notice that your intuition is sharper, or you are making better decisions. When you are connected to your Inner Wisdom, it can provide all kinds of sage advice. All you have to do is pay attention.

***Today:* Eat all your meals and snacks mindfully, meditate for thirty minutes and move mindfully for twenty-five minutes.**

***Today's Journal Question:* Describe your connection with Your Inner Wisdom as it relates to your eating habits and anything else.**

NOVEMBER 20:
MINDFUL MEDITATION REFLECTIONS

When I introduced mindful meditation to you back in January, I said that developing a practice will lead to benefits that spread to all aspects of your life. A regular meditation practice has been shown to ease chronic pain, reduce stress and anxiety, improve emotional well-being, decrease binge eating, and heal insomnia. It can also improve relationships, help your career, and enhance the overall quality of your life. So, has it? I sincerely hope it has. My wish for you is that over the course of our time together, you have benefited in ways that go beyond a different relationship with food. I want you to feel as if your whole life has improved in one way or another.

Take some time today to reflect upon your meditation practice. Think about where you were when we first started and where you are now. Consider the ways in which you are calmer, more centered, less stressed and how those changes have positively affected your life. Notice if you are less disturbed by life's little annoyances, take more things in stride, are more empathic or compassionate towards others. Are you more creative? Has your memory improved? Do you have more self-confidence, self-awareness, and self-love? It is possible that you are a different person today than you were 11 months ago. Are you? How?

Today: **Eat all your meals and snacks mindfully, meditate for thirty minutes and move mindfully for twenty-five minutes.**

Today's Journal Question: **How has having a regular meditation practice enhanced your life overall?**

NOVEMBER 21:
HOW TUNED IN ARE YOU?

Today, I want to you to check in with how tuned in you are with your body. If you have been practicing checking not only how hungry you are but also how food (and drink) feels within your body, you are truly a mindful eater. Making the decision to pay attention in the way that mindful eating requires is a big commitment. Truthfully, most people can't be bothered. They would rather find a diet, be told what and how much to eat, and be on their way. Perhaps you were like that too. I know I was, until I wasn't. Until I truly understood that the only way to have a healthy relationship with food and be at the weight that was right for me was to give up dieting completely and embrace mindful eating, I was like the others.

Tuning into my body and giving myself time to learn how my body communicates with me was quite a challenge. But I hung in there, and I hope you did too. Becoming acquainted, and then BFFs with my Inner Wisdom was the greatest gift I have ever given myself. Maybe you feel the same. If you are not there yet, no worries. Being a mindful eater is a lifelong mission, so you still have plenty of time to get good at it. Just keep practicing.

***Today:* Eat all your meals and snacks mindfully, meditate for thirty minutes and move mindfully for twenty-five minutes.**

***Today's Journal Question:* On a scale of one to ten (one being not in touch at all and ten being BFFs with your body), how tuned in are you with your body and if you are not near a ten, what do you need to do to get closer?**

NOVEMBER 22:
THE COLORS OF THE RAINBOW

Have you ever seen the full arch of a rainbow as it hugs the sky? It is a magnificent sight. ROYGBIV is how I remember the colors—red, orange, yellow, green, blue, indigo, and violet. You know where else you will find ROYGBIV? In the produce section of your local grocer. From red apples to oranges to green broccoli to blueberries to indigo-tinted boysenberries to violet-colored Japanese eggplants, your neighborhood produce department has all the colors of the rainbow for you to choose from. If you are interested in more mindfully healthy eating habits, I have a suggestion for you: simply add more colors of the rainbow to your plate. Let me ask you something, at a typical meal, how colorful is your plate? Is it possible for you to add more color while honoring your Inner Wisdom and following your Outer Guidance? Obviously if you are allergic to strawberries don't add them to a salad, but maybe a bright red tomato can decorate your plate and mindfully feed your body? Adding more fruits and vegetables to your array of mindful food choices is an effective way to bump up the nutritional content of your meals and consequently your body.

***Today:* Eat all your meals and snacks mindfully, meditate for thirty minutes and move mindfully for twenty-five minutes.**

***Today's Journal Question:* What colors currently make up a typical day of your eating?**

NOVEMBER 23:
BRUSSEL SPROUTS MEDITATION

Tomorrow is Thanksgiving and today I am tasked with preparing the Brussels sprouts. The rest of my family is occupied with other preparations, so it is just me, two bags of Brussels sprouts and a colander. As I begin to tear open the bags, I am reminded of something the Buddhist monk Thich Nhat Hanh famously said when discussing an experience he had washing dishes. To paraphrase he said, "When washing the dishes, just wash the dishes." In other words, in this moment have all your attention on the task at hand. Alone in the kitchen I decided to do as this wise sage advised and just prepare the Brussels sprouts as I prepare the Brussels sprouts. Instead of tearing open the packaging I slowly pulled the seams apart. I took a whiff of the sprouts as they lay in the bag.

Slowly, I poured them into the colander admiring their shapes and colors. I did the same with the second bag. The colander was now brimming bright green. I picked a sprout up and looked at it closely. While I knew that a Brussels sprout is part of the cabbage family, I never paid attention before. Today, I studied these mini-versions and I observed how, like snowflakes, each sprout was different in shape, size, and color. My colander was a rainbow of different shades of green. Beautiful. Then I turned on the water to rinse them. I showered them with clean warm water. I could feel the water against my hands as I carefully tossed the sprouts to clean every spot. When I turned the water off, I watched as the drop dripped from the bottom of the colander and enjoyed the vibrant green color that glistened from the bowl. It was now time to slice the sprouts. In the past I would have found this task tedious and rushed through it.

Today, I chose to slice each sprout slowly and with a loving touch. A rhythm developed as I sliced the sprouts and placed them into a bowl. My body swayed with each slice. I was truly enjoying the moment. When I finished slicing, I set the bowl aside admiring my handiwork and feeling unexpectedly serene. The next day when the Brussels sprouts were served, I felt a sense of pride and joy as my family savored them during our festive meal. To me they tasted like the best Brussels sprouts ever made! Choose a food to prepare today and give your preparation you undivided attention. Notice if it tastes different because of the extra TLC you gave it.

Today: **Eat all your meals and snacks mindfully, meditate for thirty minutes and move mindfully for twenty-five minutes.**

Today's Journal Question: **What is it like to focus all your attention on a single task?**

NOVEMBER 24:
A MINDFUL THANKSGIVING MEAL

Thanksgiving is hands-down my favorite holiday of the year. It helps that my birthday often falls on this auspicious date. I'll be honest, one the main reasons I love this holiday is the food, especially the stuffing. OMG! When I was little, and before we knew about the danger of cooking stuffing inside the bird, my father—who, as you may recall from way back in February, was always responsible for that part of the meal—would stuff the turkey with the most delicious concoction of matzah meal, celery, onions, and broth. Yes, you read right, I wrote matzah. But boy let me tell you, it was so delicious.

As my father got older and couldn't participate as he had, my sister and I would make his famous stuffing. When dinner was served, I would fill my plate with turkey, green beans, squash, potatoes (basically whatever was served) and then the stuffing. With my plate teaming with all of goodies, I would eat and eat and eat, until I was stuffed (pun intended!). That is until I became a mindful eater. My first Thanksgiving after learning about mindful eating was an eye-opener for me. When the meal was served, instead of loading up on a little bit of everything, I went for what I wanted most—the stuffing. I helped myself to a hefty portion and dug in, licking my fork so I could get every morsel. Because I was learning about mindful eating, I checked in with myself and noticed that I felt full. I didn't need to eat anymore at this time, so I stopped.

Later in the day, when I felt hungry again, I served myself another plate, but this time I was hungry for turkey and green beans. That Thanksgiving was the first Thanksgiving when I felt good after eating. This Thanksgiving mindfully choose for yourself the foods you want to eat the most and then savor them. There is no reason to overeat on Thanksgiving when you know you can eat again whenever you get hungry.

***Today:* Eat all your meals and snacks mindfully, meditate for thirty minutes and move mindfully for twenty-five minutes.**

***Today's Journal Question:* Which foods are your favorites at Thanksgiving and how can you eat them mindfully?**

NOVEMBER 25:
THE DAY AFTER THANKSGIVING

Good morning. How ya doing? It's the day after Thanksgiving and for many it is the time to hit the stores for mega-sales. For others it a time to reach for the Pepto-Bismol and lie down. What kind of day are you having? Your answer to that question may depend on whether you were a mindful or mindless eater during yesterday's festivities. So, what happened? Did you overeat? If you did, that's okay. It's not a crime. But I would like you to take some time to think about why you ate so much. Was it because this is the only day you get to eat certain foods, so you wanted to fill up? Was it because there was tension around the table and you soothed yourself with extra pie? Or was it because it's the holidays so you get to "cheat"? If you didn't overeat; and instead, remained mindful, what was that like for you? Did people give you a hard time for your choice to eat less than they did? Were you left alone to eat what you pleased? How do you feel about yourself for choosing to have a mindful Thanksgiving? Please keep in mind that Thanksgiving is just the first of many celebrations to come. The holiday season is not a reason to go mindless.

***Today:* Eat all your meals and snacks mindfully, meditate for thirty minutes and move mindfully for twenty-five minutes.**

***Today's Journal Question:* Were you mindful or mindless during your Thanksgiving meal? Why, or why not?**

NOVEMBER 26:
OUTER GUIDANCE—WHAT ABOUT A CUPPA COFFEE?

Do you start your day with a cup of coffee or black tea? If you do and you miss a day, what happens? How does your body respond? We are a caffeinated nation. Many of us can't get through the day without our cup of joe. Now that you are mindful, pay attention to how caffeine feels in your body; what it does for your energy, mood, and sleep. There is a good chance that you have been a mindless caffeine junkie and didn't even know it. If caffeine supports you and your body in a way that serves you, you may choose to continue consuming it. But if you discover that there are negative consequences, such as an upset stomach, the jitters, insomnia, or mood swings, try going without. Be mindful of any withdrawal symptoms you may feel and adjust your caffeine intake accordingly. It may not be in your best interest to go "cold-turkey." Go at your own pace.

***Today:* Eat all your meals and snacks mindfully, meditate for thirty minutes and move mindfully for twenty-five minutes.**

***Today's Journal Question:* How does your body react to caffeine?**

NOVEMBER 27:
ANOTHER DAY IN NATURE

I have lived the past thirty-something years in Los Angeles and I love the year-round temperate climate, but I must admit that as a former New Yorker I do miss the brisk fall days and snowy winters back east. There is nothing like the cool air on my face as I walk around Central Park. Or the snow-filled driveway that morphed into snowmen and snowball fights when I was a kid. Today it happens to be raining in LA, and as soon as I finish writing this entry for you, I will go outside and take a walk. I love walking in the rain. I enjoy the puddles and the raindrops. To me, the rain feels cleansing, fresh and renewing. Today, spend some time outside. Enjoy whatever weather your part of the world is offering you. Notice how being outside affects you. Can you find the good in whatever weather awaits you? Can you appreciate Mother Nature for her miraculous seasons and glorious sights and sounds?

***Today:* Eat all your meals and snacks mindfully, meditate for thirty minutes and move mindfully for twenty-five minutes.**

***Today's Journal Question:* How does spending time in nature affect your mood and food intake?**

NOVEMBER 28:
TEACH SOMEONE MEDITATION

"They" say that the best way to learn something is to teach it. Teaching makes you an expert on the very subject you are choosing to teach. I felt that way at the end of each semester as a psychology professor. By the end of the semester, I knew more about the subject I had just finished teaching than I did when the semester started. To bolster your meditation practice and to share the gift of meditation with another, I want you to teach it to someone. Now before you object that you are just a beginner and don't really know what you are doing, I assure you, you know more than you think you do, and you certainly know more than someone who has never tried meditating. Today, approach someone who you think would enjoy a meditation practice and tell her you would like to teach her how to meditate. Share with her how you started meditating and what your practice is like. If you are unsure how to teach her, simply go back to the beginning of this journey and review the days when I taught you. It's okay to use this book as a guide. Spend some time guiding your friend through her first meditation and in so doing you will strengthen your meditation muscle without even trying.

Today: **Eat all your meals and snacks mindfully, meditate for thirty minutes and move mindfully for twenty-five minutes.**

Today's Journal Question: **Teach someone to meditate and then reflect on how doing so enhanced your own practice.**

NOVEMBER 29:

THREE SQUARES A DAY

Are you still eating three square meals a day? Is your food still clock and meal dependent, or are you your own clock now? It is possible that your Inner Wisdom guides you to eat three times a day around the same times that we traditionally eat our meals. Or it is possible that your Inner Wisdom has a completely different schedule, and you find yourself eating at various times throughout the day. In fact, when you are tuned into your Inner Wisdom you may eat at different times on different days. I notice this most for me in the mornings. Some mornings I wake up hungry and before I even lace up my sneakers for a morning walk, I eat something. Other mornings, I am not hungry at all and may not feel hunger for several hours. In addition, sometimes I am hungry for a lot of food and other times, a few bites are all I need. If I were still tied to some diet plan, I would be eating in accordance with its schedule, not my own. How far have you come with your Inner Wisdom skills? If you are still struggling, that's okay. Do the best you can, when you can and the rest of the time be kind to yourself.

Today: **Eat all your meals and snacks mindfully, meditate for thirty minutes and move mindfully for twenty-five minutes.**

Today's Journal Question: **Does your eating reflect the clock on your wall or the clock in your body?**

NOVEMBER 30:
THE SCALE REVISITED

We haven't talked much about weight and scales on this journey for a reason. The journey to becoming a mindful eater is about so much more than the numbers on the scale. I'm sure you know that by now. Still, that being said, where are you in relationship with your scale? If you are like many people I work with, the scale is now an afterthought. You are so tuned with your body that you know pretty much know how much you weigh without needing to look. In fact, the number may have become irrelevant to you by now. Or not. Hopefully if you are using the scale, you are doing so as friend not foe and your scale is merely a tool on your journey and not a weapon of self-hate or disappointment. Reflect on the role the scale is playing in your life now and whether or not it serves your best interests.

Today: **Eat all your meals and snacks mindfully, meditate for thirty minutes and move mindfully for twenty-five minutes.**

Today's Journal Question: **How has your relationship with your scale changed since we began this journey?**

DECEMBER

◆◆◆

DECEMBER 1:
HOLIDAY STRESS EATING

Thanksgiving is behind us and we addressed the potential for overeating at that holiday. The truth is 'tis the season to over-indulge. At least that is what we tell ourselves. But not if you are a mindful eater. You have a choice. So, why do people overeat during the holidays? In a very non-scientific way, I have deduced three reasons for all that food: (1) it's there. Foods that are usually kept out of one's home finds its way in via gift baskets or hand-delivered homemade treats. The same is true in our offices. In fact, offices can be even worse. Having all this food around makes it easy to mindlessly eat; (2) we give ourselves permission to gorge ourselves, making promises of New Year's Resolutions and gym memberships for Christmas. This is the same as the "I'll start on Monday" refrain that precedes most diet attempts. If you are going to give yourself permission to overdo it, own that decision. Make it a conscious, mindful choice rather than an "I'll look at it later" proposition; and (3) the holidays are stressful. In my clinical practice, I made it a habit not to take vacation in December because that was often the time some of my clients needed me the most. Anticipated visits to or from relatives can spike distress. Being strapped for cash or feeling obligated to give gifts can also be part of the dilemma. If you recognize that you are stress eating over the holidays, engage in different ways to deal with the stress (my previous books can really help here). Of course, I want you to enjoy the holidays including all the goodies offered—not just all of them or all at once. Think about your choices. Check in with your body and if stress is the reason you overeat, increase your meditation to ease the pain.

***Today:* Eat all your meals and snacks mindfully, meditate for thirty minutes and move mindfully for thirty minutes.**

***Today's Journal Question:* What role does stress play in your food choices over the holiday season?**

DECEMBER 2:
ADDRESSING CHALLENGES

As we settle into the last month of our year together, we will spend some time reviewing key concepts and skills, so you can feel confident as you move ahead into the next year. I have said many times that mindful eating is a process and its goal is not perfection. For me the goals of mindful eating are balance, peace of mind and being comfortable in my own skin. Keeping these goals in mind, how are you faring? Are you feeling challenged anywhere? Are you stuck somehow? Changing a lifetime of habits is not going to happen overnight. That fact is in part why I wrote this book as a yearlong journey. Here is a list of the major concepts, skills and tools we have been exploring. Look them over, and if there are any you feel wobbly about, go back through these pages and begin again: Inner Wisdom; Outer Guidance; Meditation Practice; Mindful Hunger, Thirst, Fullness and Satisfaction; Mindless and Emotional Eating; Gratitude; and Self-Compassion. Remember, this isn't a race. This is your life we are talking about so take your time and, most important, be kind to yourself.

***Today:* Eat all your meals and snacks mindfully, meditate for thirty minutes and move mindfully for thirty minutes.**

***Today's Journal Question:* What aspects of mindful eating do you need to review and keep working at?**

DECEMBER 3:
DEEPENING YOUR MEDITATION PRACTICE

The central component of this mindful eating approach is meditation. Meditation is what separates this method from other non-diet efforts. Throughout the year you have been building a solid practice. By slowly increasing the time you meditate over several months, you had a chance to develop the habit of meditating. My intention was to help you establish a thirty-minute-a-day practice. If you are not here yet, no worries. Keep sitting and lengthening the time you sit at a pace that feels right for you. If 30 minutes will always feel too long, go shorter. Just keep at it. A daily practice of any length is better than a spotty practice of longer duration. If you have reached the thirty-minute threshold, you can decide to deepen your practice if you want to.

For example, you can choose to stop doing guided meditations and meditate in silence. You can meditate twice a day and/or lengthen your sitting time. You can choose to join a meditation group or attend silent retreats. You can explore different forms of meditation beyond mindfulness-based meditation to enhance your experience. Make your practice whatever you want it to be. Allow it to evolve in any way that serves you best. You cannot do this wrong. Just keep at it.

Today: **Eat all your meals and snacks mindfully, meditate for thirty minutes and move mindfully for thirty minutes.**

Today's Journal Question: **How can you deepen your meditation practice?**

DECEMBER 4:

ARE SUGARPLUM FAIRIES DANCING IN YOUR HEAD?

One aspect of mindful eating that still totally fascinates me is the images of food that pop into my head as my body starts to get hungry. It happened again today. It had been several hours since I had breakfast and I noticed some of my hunger signals—slight grumbling in my stomach, less ability to concentrate. I wanted to finish what I was reading before I prepared my food, but my mind wouldn't let me. As hard as I tried to stay focused on the words in front of me, my mind kept showing me a cantaloupe. Juicy, shiny wedges of light orange shimmered in my head. Then my mind shifted to the cantaloupe I had ripening on the counter. I could no longer read. I knew it was time to cut that melon and serve myself some slices. So, I put down my book, and mindfully cut and ate my cantaloupe. I ate about 1/3 of the melon and felt full and satisfied. I cleared my plate and went back to my book. This time, I could concentrate once again. Most of the time the food images that appear in my head are exactly the right food for that moment. If I don't have that exact food, I either go get it or mindfully choose something that is a close second.

Today: **Eat all your meals and snacks mindfully, meditate for thirty minutes and move mindfully for thirty minutes.**

Today's Journal Question: **If food images pop into your head when you are hungry, what do you do?**

DECEMBER 5:
REVISITING MINDFUL HUNGER

This afternoon as I sat down to prepare this passage for you, I found myself unable to concentrate. My focus kept wandering off the page. Then I noticed it—the rumbling in my stomach. I was hungry. For me, a typical hunger signal is loss of focus. So, I had a choice to make. I could power through and keep writing or I could acknowledge my need to eat and take a break. I chose the break. I got up from my computer and reached into the insulated bag I carry with me. Inside I found a protein bar. I have learned that these bars are good for me when I am hungry and either don't have time for a "proper" snack or when I know I want to be hungry again soon because of plans I made.

Today, I knew that I would be eating my dinner soon but still wanted to address the hunger I had now. The protein bar was a perfect choice. I stepped away from my computer and sat on my couch. I unwrapped the protein bar and ate it. It took about five minutes and I was done. I returned to my computer better able to finish the writing I had started. I share this little anecdote to remind you how mindful hunger works. I was able to recognize not only my need to eat but also what and how much would suit me best. How are you doing with this skill? Are you able to recognize your hunger signals? Are you tuned into your body now? If not, why not? Spend some time revisiting how your body shares the news that it's hunger with you. Keep practicing until you and your hunger are on good terms.

***Today:* Eat all your meals and snacks mindfully, meditate for thirty minutes and move mindfully for thirty minutes.**

***Today's Journal Question:* How does hunger show up for you?**

DECEMBER 6:
REVISITING MINDFUL FULLNESS

Equally important to knowing your hunger signals is knowing your fullness signals. Being able to stop eating when you are full is how you will reduce to and stay at the weight that is right for you. How are you doing with this skill? Can you identify when you have had enough to meet your body's nutritional needs? Are you able to stop? What helped me be able to stop was knowing that I will be able to eat again the next time I am hungry, and if I don't eat more than I need now, that moment will come sooner rather than later. I know I am full when I start to lose interest in the food. When I start to question why I am still eating. For me fullness is a pleasant sensation under my belly button. Not too much, not too little, just right. Am I perfect with recognizing and acting on my fullness? No, I don't know anybody who is. What I do know is that the more I honor my fullness the better I feel.

***Today:* Eat all your meals and snacks mindfully, meditate for thirty minutes and move mindfully for thirty minutes.**

***Today's Journal Question:* How are you doing recognizing and acting on your signs of fullness?**

DECEMBER 7:
REVISITING MINDFUL SATISFACTION

Ah, so good! The sigh of satisfaction. It may come after you meet a deadline at work, take the first sip of your favorite Chardonnay, cross the finish line at a 10K, or when you bite into Aunt Selma's homemade apple pie. Satisfaction is an important part of mindful eating and the one I appreciate the most. We need to be satisfied when we eat, or we will keep looking for something else to eat. That can lead to grazing, which can lead to excess weight. Before I became a mindful eater, I would eat foods that I didn't particularly like. String cheese, not my fav. Grilled chicken breasts, no thank you. Why did I eat foods that I didn't really care for? Because I thought eating them was part of a healthy diet. Because I thought I was supposed to. As a mindful eater I gave myself permission to eat foods that I enjoy, not just those that are "good for me." What about you? Have you given yourself permission to eat foods that taste satisfying to you?

Taste satisfaction worked another way for me too. Once I started eating mindfully, I brought foods into my home that I had previously kept out because I thought they were "forbidden." Then I tested these foods. When I was hungry, I served myself a serving and approached eating mindfully. I slowly ate my portion, tasting each bite and you know what? Some of my previously forbidden foods were not favorites after all. Who would guess that mac and cheese can be too greasy or a glazed donut too sweet? Once I really started to taste my food, I naturally gravitated towards foods that I prefer. For me, being able to eat only foods that truly taste good has been the biggest contributor to my success as a mindful eater. How about you?

***Today:* Eat all your meals and snacks mindfully, meditate for thirty minutes and move mindfully for thirty minutes.**

Today's Journal Question: **What is it like (or what would it be like) to give yourself permission to eat only foods that truly tasted good to you?**

DECEMBER 8:
REVISITING MINDFUL CHOICES

As we come close to the end of your first year of mindful eating, I hope that you understand that mindful eating is all about choice. By paying attention to how you feel, what your body needs, and how food affects you, you are giving yourself information to help you make the most informed decisions about what, when and how much to eat at any given time. No food is off-limits (unless medically restricted), so you can enjoy anything you like when you do so mindfully. And even if you slip back into mindless eating for a meal, a day, or a month, you always have the choice to begin again. Choice is power. Mindful eating is a powerful way to make peace with food and your weight struggles. What choice will you make today?

Today: **Eat all your meals and snacks mindfully, meditate for thirty minutes and move mindfully for thirty minutes.**

Today's Journal Question: **How have your choices changed over the past eleven months?**

DECEMBER 9:
REVISITING GRATITUDE

During this time of year, it is wonderful to take stock of everything you have to be grateful for. Even if you feel harried by holiday shopping, overwhelmed by all the invitations you have received, or impatient trying to wrangle the kids for a road trip, there is always something to appreciate. Stopping to notice all that is good amid chaos is being mindful. Saying thank you to those you encounter on any given day is being mindful. Feeling joy for the smallest detail is being mindful. Being and expressing gratitude is being mindful. And being and expressing gratitude changes how you feel which in turn may change how you eat.

Today: **Eat all your meals and snacks mindfully, meditate for thirty minutes and move mindfully for thirty minutes.**

Today's Journal Question: **Make a list of ten things you are grateful for and why you are grateful for them.**

DECEMBER 10:
A MINDFUL BATH

Amidst the holiday rush it is important to take time for yourself. It is so easy to get distracted from self-care when there are gifts to wrap, trees to trim and candles to light. One way I like to relax during the holiday season is with a luxurious mindful bath. What makes a bath mindful? Intention does. Set an intention to set aside a half-hour or so for yourself. Set an intention to be completely left alone—no cell phones, no knocks on the bathroom door. You get the idea. And set an intention to make the bath as lovely as possible. Make bubbles. Drop in essential oils. Light scented candles. Play music. Burn incense. Do whatever you would like to feel soothed while in your bath. If you don't have access to a bathtub, you can do the same thing with a long, hot shower. The key is to make time to pamper yourself. You deserve it.

Today: **Eat all your meals and snacks mindfully, meditate for thirty minutes and move mindfully for thirty minutes.**

Today's Journal Question: **If you were to take mindful bath or shower, what would you do to make it special?**

DECEMBER 11:
TAKE A PENNY, GIVE A PENNY

Have you ever seen one of those jars on a countertop that says, "Take a Penny, Give a Penny"? If you have you know that the jar is there so people who pay cash for something don't have to struggle finding a cent if they need it. The jar reflects our honor system and supports the idea that we can share with each other without greed or sacrifice. We can do the same with food. We are in the holiday season and, sadly, some families do not have money for a holiday meal. Now is the time for you to offer compassion and generosity to those in need. Whether you donate time or money, find a way to share yourself and your food with others. Mindful living is steeped in kindness, interconnectedness, and gratitude.

There is no better way to demonstrate these tenets than by making sure someone has enough food to eat. Each month I make a small donation to a local charity that feeds children in my community. While the donation amount is small, the benefits are huge. I am so blessed to always have (more than) enough food that I think it is imperative upon me to help those who don't. Find a way to feed another and you will engage in a beautifully mindful act.

Today: **Eat all your meals and snacks mindfully, meditate for thirty minutes and move mindfully for thirty minutes.**

Today's Journal Question: **How can you offer food to someone in need?**

DECEMBER 12:
MINDFUL GIFT-GIVING

If giving gifts is part of your holiday tradition, I would like to show you how to select those gifts in a mindful manner. To begin, think about the recipient of the gift. Who is she? What does she enjoy? Ask yourself, what would this person want? So often we choose gifts based on what we want for them rather than what they would want for themselves. Spend some time thinking before shopping and your selection will most likely improve. Another way to give a gift is to give a gift of your time. I'm sure the overworked single mom on your gift list could use someone to do a chore for her rather than a new sweater. Your sister-in-law who complains she and her husband never get out would probably love an offer to babysit in place of a blender. When you take the time to be mindful of who your gift recipient is, what their needs are, and what they might appreciate the most, your gift-giving should be much easier. And if you feel pressure to get the perfect gift, give yourself the gift of releasing that pressure. There truly is no such thing as perfection anyway, so why bother?

Today: **Eat all your meals and snacks mindfully, meditate for thirty minutes and move mindfully for thirty minutes.**

Today's Journal Question: **What kind of gifts of time can you give your loved ones this season?**

DECEMBER 13:
MINDFUL HOLIDAY SHOPPING

If you close your eyes and listen, I bet you can imagine hearing sidewalk Santas ringing their bells and carolers singing their favorite tune. If you close your eyes, I bet you can imagine smelling the pine from the Christmas trees and the oil from the Hanukkah pancakes. But when you open your eyes, I bet you are met with a long list of tasks to do, the least of which is holiday shopping. If holiday shopping makes you anxious, don't fret. You can engage in mindful shopping and enjoy yourself. To shop mindfully simply slow down and take your time. Don't rush around like a rabbit being chased by a greyhound. Instead, choose to enjoy the sounds, smells, and sights of the season. In less than three weeks, it'll all be gone so, relish it now. If you feel as if you are running around too much, stop for a few minutes several times a day and just breathe. Wherever you are, stop, get centered, and take your breaths. Do this as many times as you need to. Two or three deep breaths can do wonders to calm a holiday-frenzied mind.

***Today:* Eat all your meals and snacks mindfully, meditate for thirty minutes and move mindfully for thirty minutes.**

***Today's Journal Question:* How can you take a few breathing breaks during this hectic time?**

DECEMBER 14:
ANNUAL CHECKUP

This morning I went for my annual mammogram. I get this exam as part of my health regimen. While I was waiting for the doctor, I thought about the last time I was here and what I had accomplished in the past year. To start with, this time last year I had only recently completed by training as an MB-EAT Instructor and was imagining the creation of TAME Your Appetite: The Art of Mindful Eating. I was also a newbie to meditation and mindful eating and was struggling to find my way. Now, a year later TAME is up and running and mindful eating and meditation are everyday occurrences for me. Then, I thought about where I would like to be next year when I return for my mammogram.

I imagined this book being in the hands of a publisher, my TAME programs gaining momentum and my being even healthier than I am today. What about you? Where were you this time last year? What have you accomplished, learned and experienced? There is value in staying aware of where we are, where we've been and where we are going. Choose an annual day or event that you can use as a benchmark to review your life. How about today?

***Today:* Eat all your meals and snacks mindfully, meditate for thirty minutes and move mindfully for thirty minutes.**

***Today's Journal Question:* Describe what your life was like one year ago, how it is today and what you might like to have be true in a year.**

DECEMBER 15:

TAKEAWAYS

You've got two weeks to go and you will have spent an entire year studying, practicing and becoming a mindful eater. What have you learned? What about you and your life are different now? How has this journey changed you? Besides school, have you ever spent this much consistent time and energy on any one task? If you had to put into words what this year meant to you, what would you say? What are the most significant things that you can take with you from this journey into the rest of your life? Better self-awareness? Peace with food? A meditation practice? A calmer disposition? Tools for coping with life that don't include food? All the above? Today, reflect on your journey and think about what were the most important lessons, accomplishments and challenges that define this year.

***Today:* Eat all your meals and snacks mindfully, meditate for thirty minutes and move mindfully for thirty minutes.**

***Today's Journal Question:* What can you take away from this journey?**

DECEMBER 16:

EIGHT DAYS OF MINDFULNESS

In celebration of Hanukkah, I would like to offer eight days of mindfulness. Here are eight mindful tips for the next eight days.

Mindful Tip 1: Every bite is an opportunity to practice mindful eating.

Mindful Tip 2: Mindfulness is simply being present with purpose and intention.

Mindful Tip 3: A quick body scan can center you, regroup your thoughts and release stress. A few minutes a day can do wonders for you. Give it a try.

Mindful Tip 4: Be grateful today for everything that happens—everything!

Mindful Tip 5: Decide what you are really hungry for and then provide it for yourself. There is no better healing than that.

Mindful Tip 6: Feeling off? Take a walk. Get some oxygen flowing and before you know it, you'll be in the flow too.

Mindful Tip 7: Appreciate yourself today. Acknowledge yourself for something wonderful that you did. You deserve it.

Mindful Tip 8: Want to learn self-compassion? Make a list of three things you did well each day.

Today: **Eat all your meals and snacks mindfully, meditate for thirty minutes and move mindfully for thirty minutes.**

Today's Journal Question: **Make a list of your favorite mindful tips.**

DECEMBER 17:
WEIGHT LOSS REVISITED

Like with the scale, we haven't talked much about your actual weight on this journey. By now you know that becoming a mindful eater is about so much more than how much you weigh or how much weight you have lost. If you are like many people I work with, by the time you have come this far in your journey, weight loss is no longer the focal point. I hope that your relationship with food and your weight has developed in such a way that you are reaching the weight that is right for you with little or no effort. Reflect on how you feel about your weight and using mindful eating as your way to manage your weight. If you have reached the weight that is right for you, congratulations. Continue to use mindfulness to maintain. If you have not reached it, keep going. The more mindful you are, the closer you will get to your goal.

Today: **Eat all your meals and snacks mindfully, meditate for thirty minutes and move mindfully for thirty minutes.**

Today's Journal Question: **Where are you on your weight-loss path?**

DECEMBER 18:

HAVE YOU MASTERED QUALITY OVER QUANTITY?

I've got a question for you. Be honest, are you truly eating foods you like? Or do you still find yourself making choices based on what you think you should eat? My hope is that, by now, you have discovered the value of eating what you really want and enjoy. I hope, too, that you have discovered that by eating foods you really want, you feel more satisfied and that eating satisfying food leads to eating less. For me, I think this was the secret to my success. By giving myself permission to eat the foods I wanted, not the foods I thought I should eat, I lost my excess weight. I found that by making those choices, I naturally ate less. No deliberately cutting portions. No intentionally choosing low-fat this or sugar-free that, unless those were my preferred choices, and sometimes they were. It took a while, but I feel I mastered the "quality over quantity" principle of mindful eating. Have you?

Today: **Eat all your meals and snacks mindfully, meditate for thirty minutes and move mindfully for thirty minutes.**

Today's Journal Question: **Are you eating more for quality, and if so, how has that affected your portion sizes and your weight?**

DECEMBER 19:

EQUANIMITY REVISITED

At the end of January, I introduced you to the concept of equanimity. Now, the middle of the holiday season, may be a good time to revisit it. The term equanimity has its origins in Latin and means "to be even in mind." When you are in a state of equanimity, you can keep it together even in the midst of chaos. You are not unconcerned or unsympathetic to what is going on around you, rather, you are peacefully observant. You make the choice not to be distressed by what is happening and, instead, you choose to be centered and calm. To get to that centered, calm place, repeat these phrases in meditation: "May I be balanced. May I be at peace. May I accept things as they are. May I accept myself just as I am." You can also replace the word "I" with anyone or anything else that serves your needs.

Today: **Eat all your meals and snacks mindfully, meditate for thirty minutes and move mindfully for thirty minutes.**

Today's Journal Question: **How can meditating repeating the equanimity**

phrases above help you get through the rest of the holiday season?

DECEMBER 20:
ARE YOU A GOURMET YET?

By now, as mindful eating is becoming more second-nature to you, you may have noticed that you have become a picky eater, choosing only the best and discarding what you do not want or like. I'd like to share with you a story about bad potato salad. There is a shop in my city that sells delicious, homemade potato salad with only whole natural ingredients. Whenever I find myself in that shop, I buy some. Last week was no exception. I bought the potato salad, placed it in my refrigerator and promptly forgot about it. That happens now. Since my mind no longer strategizes what I will eat and when I will eat it, I forget. Today, I found myself getting hungry, so I checked in with my Inner Wisdom for guidance on what I should eat. The potato salad came to mind.

Usually when I eat the potato salad, I have some sort of sandwich with it. But today, I didn't want a sandwich. I wanted a scoop of the potato salad with a scoop of chicken salad on a bed of lettuce. I prepared my plate, sat down to eat it and after a few moments of centering and mindful thinking, I put a forkful of the potato salad into my mouth anticipating its creamy, delicious flavor. Instead, what I got was a tart, somewhat acidic taste. I spit the disappointing forkful into a napkin and sighed. I got up from the table to retrieve the salad's carton and discovered that it was past its "eat by" date. Oops. (I guess I was mindless by not reading the label before I served myself the scoop.) I went back to my plate and checked in again with my Inner Wisdom. Sure, I could eat the tart salad, or I could make another choice. My Inner Wisdom guided me to throw the potato salad out, scoop another serving of the chicken salad over my lettuce and enjoy my lunch. And enjoy I did. I love being a picky eater. Food tastes so much better that way.

***Today:* Eat all your meals and snacks mindfully, meditate for thirty minutes and move mindfully for thirty minutes.**

***Today's Journal Question:* How have your eating preferences changed over this year? Are you a picky eater or gourmet?**

DECEMBER 21:
DO YOU STILL EMOTIONALLY EAT?

On a scale of one to ten, how much emotional eating do you still do? One being "only occasionally" and ten being "it's still a big problem, help me!" Before learning about and teaching mindful eating, my area of expertise was emotional eating. Having used M&M's to get through law school, I know a thing or two about emotional eating. I have said this before and it is worth repeating now, it is not a crime to emotionally eat. Everybody does it and I mean everybody. Whoever tells you they don't most likely doesn't understand what emotional eating is. If you meet such a person, tell them that emotional eating is eating when you are not physically hungry. See, everybody does it. So, back to my question: On a scale of one to ten, how much emotional eating do you still do?

How about another question: Compared to how much emotional eating you did before you learned mindful eating, on a scale of one to ten, how much emotional eating do you still do? It is my hope that by now you understand the difference between physical and emotional hunger, are in tune with your Inner Wisdom, are maintaining a meditation practice, and are finding other ways to cope. If you are still struggling, it's okay. Growth is a process. Remember after every binge or emotional eating event, you can always begin again (we will look at "beginning again" again tomorrow). If you want more help, check out my previous books, *Do You Use Food to Cope?* and The Best Diet Begins in Your Mind. The store on the TAMEYourAppetite.com website also has audio and visual tools you can use. Meanwhile, do what you can without judgment or ridicule, be kind to yourself and practice self-compassion. Ending emotional eating is not easy, give yourself a break.

Today: **Eat all your meals and snacks mindfully, meditate for thirty minutes and move mindfully for thirty minutes.**

Today's Journal Question: **Describe your emotional eating habits now and this time last year.**

DECEMBER 22:
BEGIN AGAIN WITH BEGINNER'S MIND

Yesterday I reminded you that if you find yourself emotionally eating, you can always begin again eating mindfully with your very next bite. In mindfulness, you can always begin again with whatever you do. Fell off the meditation wagon? Begin again. Eating in front of the computer? Begin again. Ignoring Outer Guidance? Begin again. Silencing your Inner Wisdom? Begin again. Back in April, I introduced the idea of beginner's mind to you. To remind you, the idea of a having a "beginner's mind" comes to us from Zen Buddhism. When you have a "beginner's mind," you approach whatever is in front of you with openness, newness, and eagerness as if you were brand new to the subject or task at hand and are ready to learn.

The Buddhists tell us to always come to life with a beginner's mind. When you do, you leave behind any presumptions, judgments and biases and see what's in front of you with fresh eyes. Think of a child the first time she sees snow. Or how you felt when you traveled to a different culture and witnessed something you had never seen before. With a beginner's mind, life is curious, adventurous and intriguing. Try approaching this journey, any problem you may have, or difficulty you face with a beginner's mind and see what happens.

***Today:* Eat all your meals and snacks mindfully, meditate for thirty minutes and move mindfully for thirty minutes.**

Today's Journal Question: What can you experience with a beginner's mind?

DECEMBER 23:
"WHAT IF" REVISITED?

When we began our journey together, I asked you the question Dr. Jean Kristeller asks, "What if a year from now you lost weight, maybe not as much as you'd like, but you were more in control of your life and eating and the weight you lost felt permanent because it reflected change you could live with for the rest of your life?" You are a week away from the one-year mark, so, what happened? Where are you in your weight-loss journey? Has your relationship with food changed? Do you feel as if whatever weight you lost is gone for good? I hope so. I hope that upon reflection you can see the improvements I wanted for you when we first began.

***Today:* Eat all your meals and snacks mindfully, meditate for thirty minutes and move mindfully for thirty minutes.**

***Today's Journal Question:* Reflect on this passing year and whether you have lost weight, if you feel were more in control of your life and eating,**

and whether whatever weight you lost feels permanent.

DECEMBER 24:

MINDFUL EVES

The day or period of time immediately before a holiday, event or special occasion is called an "eve." Today is Christmas Eve and whether you celebrate Christmas or not, let's take moment to think about the eves in your life and how you might celebrate them mindfully. What eves do you have? New Year's Eve? Halloween Eve? The eve before your birthday, anniversary, first day of school? An eve is anticipatory. You know that tomorrow something wonderful will happen. When we are mindful of an eve it means that we are aware that the eve exists too. We live in this moment, not just the big day. Being mindful means being aware and being present. Acknowledging an eve means that you are in the present not the future. What wonderful things can an eve offer? Which eves can you be present for?

***Today:* Eat all your meals and snacks mindfully, meditate for thirty minutes and move mindfully for thirty minutes.**

***Today's Journal Question:* Name three things about an eve that you can be mindful of.**

DECEMBER 25:

MINDFUL MERRY CHRISTMAS

Worried that you will overdo it on holiday ham or sweet apple pie? Don't. Use your mindful eating skills and you will enjoy this Christmas more than any other. Remember, slow down, tune into your body, choose the foods you want the most, savor each bite, and stop when you are comfortably full knowing that you can eat again when you are hungry later. Don't want to be mindful this Christmas? Rather go mindless? That's your choice. If you choose to be mindless, remember to be conscious about your decision. Own it and tomorrow plan on returning to your mindful eating habits.

***Today:* Eat all your meals and snacks mindfully, meditate for thirty minutes and move mindfully for thirty minutes.**

Today's Journal Question: **Which mindful eating skills will you use to have a very merry Christmas?**

DECEMBER 26:
MINDFUL INTENTIONS

As we approach the end of our year together, it is time to explore what your intentions will be going forward. An intention is a determination to act in a certain way or to pursue a particular goal or experience. With respect to mindful eating, your intention could be to become more comfortable leaving food on your plate when you know that you are full, to use meditation to ease emotional distress, to continue your meditation practice, or repeat this year in order to strengthen your habits. To make your intention more than a mere statement on a page, follow up your intention with some sort of action.

For example, if you want to continue with your meditation practice, buy a journal in which you can record your sessions. To make sure your action isn't just one more thing to do, follow up your action with observations. For example, if you find yourself resisting getting another journal to record your meditation practice, why? Or maybe you rush out to pick up a new beautiful one, why that action? Explore your actions with neutral, non-judgmental observations. Then, follow up your observations with a mindful choice about what to do next.

Today: **Eat all your meals and snacks mindfully, meditate for thirty minutes and move mindfully for thirty minutes.**

Today's Journal Question: **What intention(s) do you have for the coming year?**

DECEMBER 27:
ANOTHER MINDFUL RAISIN

Remember back in January you began your mindful eating journey with the raisin exercise? Today let's do it again. Grab a raisin (or some other morsel of food if you don't like raisins) and begin:

- Put the raisin (or morsel of food) on a fork, spoon or between your fingers.

- Look at it. Notice its colors and textures.
- Bring it to your nose and sniff. Notice its scent.
- Touch it to your lips. Feel its texture.
- Place it in your mouth, but don't chew. Feel it. Roll it over your tongue.
- Bite into it. Notice its flavor.
- Chew it but don't swallow.
- Now swallow and feel the food slip down your throat.
- Place your hand on your stomach and imagine the bite of food settling there.

How was it? By repeating this exercise can you see how far you have come with your mindful eating? Think back to that first day and reflect on how getting started with a single bite like this taught you to become a mindful eater. It's been a great journey, hasn't it? Congratulations!

***Today:* Eat all your meals and snacks mindfully, meditate for thirty minutes and move mindfully for thirty minutes.**

***Today's Journal Question:* How was eating the raisin mindfully today different than when you did it back in January?**

DECEMBER 28:

GETTING READY TO MOVE ON

This is it. We are winding down. In three days, our year-long journey together will come to an end. As we get ready to move on, here's a simple summary of seven basic skills for mindful eating which you can keep handy. When you prepare to eat something remember to do the following: (1) take a moment and get centered, breathe, and focus your attention on this eating "event"; (2) check in with your hunger and fullness feelings, noting them silently to yourself; (3) observe the food you have chosen to eat, noticing what it looks like, feels like, and smells like; (4) think about all that it took to get this food to you, consider the farmers, manufacturers, transportation vehicles, stock clerks, and cashiers, and silently thank them for their participation; (5) eat your food slowly, paying attention to how it tastes and feels in your mouth, noticing when or if the taste changes; (6) check in again with your hunger and fullness signals, noticing what has changed; and (7) finish eating when you notice that you are comfortably full.

***Today:* Eat all your meals and snacks mindfully, meditate for thirty minutes and move mindfully for thirty minutes.**

***Today's Journal Question:* How do you feel about moving on from our work together?**

DECEMBER 29:

MOVING ON AND REMAINING MINDFUL

As we move on, I want to encourage you to continue living a mindful life. It is not necessary to be mindful of everything, that's impossible, but the more you choose to be mindful, the fuller and richer your life can become. In her landmark book, *Mindfulness*, author and social psychologist Ellen J. Lange talks about second-order mindfulness which is choosing what to be mindful about. She acknowledges that we cannot be mindful of everything, but as she writes, "we can always be mindful of something." She goes on to remind us that "mindful awareness of different options gives us greater control," and that "rather than being a chore, mindfulness engages us in a continuing momentum."

Simple ways to continue the momentum of mindfulness regardless of what you are doing are: (1) stay in the present moment, when your mind wanders to the past or future gently bring it back to the here-and-now; (2) slow down when you catch yourself speeding through an activity; (3) do one thing at a time, multi-task only when absolutely necessary; (4) continue to eat mindfully as best you can; (5) maintain your meditation practice, trying to sit for a least a few minutes every day; and (6) remember that whatever happens you can always begin again.

***Today:* Eat all your meals and snacks mindfully, meditate for thirty minutes and move mindfully for thirty minutes.**

***Today's Journal Question:* How can you continue to live a mindful life in the months and years to come?**

DECEMBER 30:

MINDFUL GOALS FOR THE COMING YEAR

I am a goal-setter. I have filled notebooks, planners and journals with goals. Some of my goals repeat year after year, such as travel more, sleep better, spend more time with family and friends. Others I fulfill and gleefully check off, like finishing a marathon or becoming a mindful eater. Still more, many, many, more, get written down and then forgotten. Oh well. No worries. No judgment. I just start again. Using the intentions you wrote about on December 26, create some goals for the upcoming year. Make them simple or audacious. Your choice. Write them in a notebook, day planner, journal, postcard, bulletin board, vision board, or anywhere else that suits you. If you like you can use these goals as a guide for the coming year or not. In whatever way you choose to use the goals you have created, be mindful of why you chose them and what you are doing with them.

***Today:* Eat all your meals and snacks mindfully, meditate for thirty minutes and move mindfully for thirty minutes.**

***Today's Journal Question:* Use today to write down your mindful goals for next year.**

DECEMBER 31:
ENDING THE YEAR MINDFULLY

Congratulations! You are at the end of our year's journey to mindful eating. Now it is time to celebrate your success. Think about where you were when you started. What did a typical day look like food-wise? How attentive were you to your eating? How much of your eating was ruled by diets or binges? Were you a mindless eater? How much mindless eating do you do now? How much emotional eating? Early in the year I asked you, "What if a year from now you lost weight, maybe not as much as you'd like, but you were more in control of your life and eating and the weight you lost felt permanent because it reflected change you could live with for the rest of your life?" Do you remember how you answered that question? Where are you now compared to where the question suggests? I hope that you have experienced growth in your relationship with food. If you are not yet where you want to be, repeat this journey. Follow the 365 entries again. Add to what you have already achieved by doing more. Or, if you prefer, choose your favorite meditations, tools and techniques and hone them. The more you practice the greater your success.

Today: Eat all your meals and snacks mindfully, meditate for thirty minutes and move mindfully for thirty minutes.

Today's Journal Question: Describe this year's journey to mindful eating.

◆◆◆

♦♦♦

Thank You!

I want to thank you for taking this journey with me. In many ways, your journey is just starting. Your relationship with food is ever evolving. If you would like me to be part of your continuing journey, follow my blog on my website TAMEYourAppetite.com and join my communities on Facebook, Twitter, LinkedIn and Instagram. If you'd like, attend a TAME Your Appetite workshop or participate in one of the TAME programs.

Whatever you do and wherever you go, I wish you peace with food.

Dr. Sheila

♦♦♦

Acknowledgments

A special thank you to Dr. Jean Kristeller and Andrea Lieberstein for their work researching, developing and teaching MB-EAT. Without your work, guidance and mentorship I would not be an MB-EAT instructor.

I also want to thank my accountability partners—Madge Beletsky, Diane Currran, Gretchen Kubacky, Judy Ludy, Karen Owoc, and Deirdre O'Conner—who stood patiently in the background as I toiled away to take my mindful eating work to the next level. Without your help, support and unwavering faith, I would still be circling the drain. Thank you!

To my mindful meditation teachers, Natalie Bell, Celeste Young and Matthew Silverstein, thank you for helping me deepen my practice through your example.

A heartfelt thank you to Chellie Campbell, author of *The Wealthy Spirit: Daily Affirmations for Financial Stress Reduction*, whose 365 affirmations and personal stories inspired me to structure this book in the same way.

Lastly, to the clients and students who joined me in this journey and whose own stories inform this work.

About the Author

Dr. Sheila Forman holds a Ph.D. in Psychology and practiced psychotherapy for over twenty years before becoming a Mindfulness-Based Eating Awareness Training (MB-EAT) Instructor. For her entire career, Dr. Sheila has been helping people address weight and food issues by teaching how to cope with emotions without overeating and, more recently, how to eliminate mindless eating with mindfulness meditation and other mindful skills and techniques.

Her program, *TAME Your Appetite – The Art of Mindful Eating,* is a non-diet approach to weight management, incorporating all that Dr. Sheila knows about healing emotional and mindless eating.

For more information about *TAME*, go to TAMEYourAppetite.com or email Dr. Sheila at Info@TAMEYourAppetite.com.

Additional Resources

APPS

Calm
Headspace
Insight Timer

BOOKS

Books by Dr. Sheila

Do You Use Food to Cope? A Comprehensive 15-Week Program for Overcoming Emotional Overeating published by Writer's Club Press, 2002.

Manage Your Emotions, Manage Your Weight an EBook available in the store at www.TAMEYourAppetite.com.

Self-Fullness: The Art of Loving and Caring for Your "Self" published by Writer's Club Press, 2000.

Stop Dieting – Start Living an EBook available in the store at www.TAMEYourAppetite.com.

The Best Diet Begins in Your Mind: Eliminate the Eight Emotional Obstacles to Permanent Weight Loss published by iUniverse, 2015.

TAME Your Appetite: The Art of Mindful Eating published by TVGuestpert Publishing 2022.

Meditation

Mindfulness Meditation for Beginners by J. Kabat-Zinn.

Real Happiness by Sharon Salzberg published by Workman Publishing, 2011.

Soul Centered by Sarah McLean published by Hay House, Inc., 2012.

Mindfulness

A Path with Heart by Jack Kornfield published by Bantam, 1993.

Coming to Our Senses: Healing Ourselves and the World through Mindfulness by J. Kabat-Zinn published by Hyperion 2006.

Full Catastrophe Living by J. Kabat-Zinn.

Mindfulness by Ellen J. Langer, published by DeCapo Press, 1989 and 2014.

Mindfulness in Plain English by H. Gunaratana published by Wisdom Publications, 1991.

The Miracle of Mindfulness by Thich Nhat Hanh.

Touching Peace by Thich Nhat Hanh.

True Refuge: Finding Peace and Freedom in Your Own Awakened Heart by Tara Brach published by Random House, 2013.

Wherever You Are, There You Are by J. Kabat-Zinn.

WEBSITES

www.Chopracentermeditations.com

www.HayHouse.com

www.marc.ucla.edu

www.Mindfulweightcontrol.com

www.SoundsTrue.com

www.TheCenterForMindfulEating.org

Join Our Community

Become part of Dr. Sheila's mindful eating community by joining

- Her email list at TAMEYourAppetite.com
- Facebook.com/TameYourAppetite
- Twitter: DrSheila@TAMEAppetite
- Instagram: @TameYourAppetite
- DrSheilaForman@LinkedIn.com

Published by

TVGUESTPERT PUBLISHING

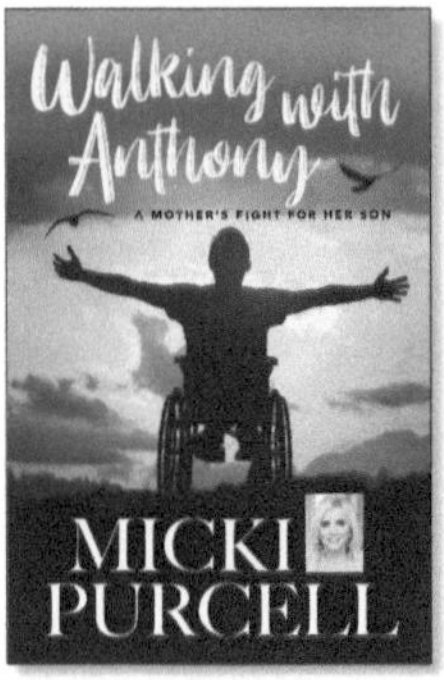

MICKI PURCELL
Walking With Anthony: A Mother's Fight For Her Son
Hardcover $22.95
Kindle: $9.99

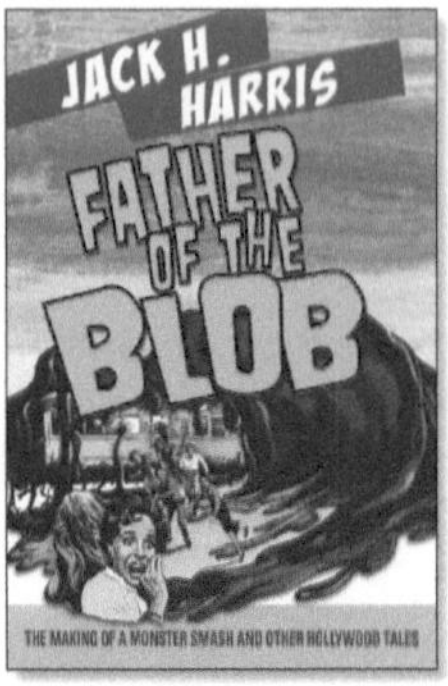

JACK H. HARRIS
Father of the Blob: The Making of a Monster Smash and Other Hollywood Tales
Paperback: $16.95
Kindle/Nook: $9.99

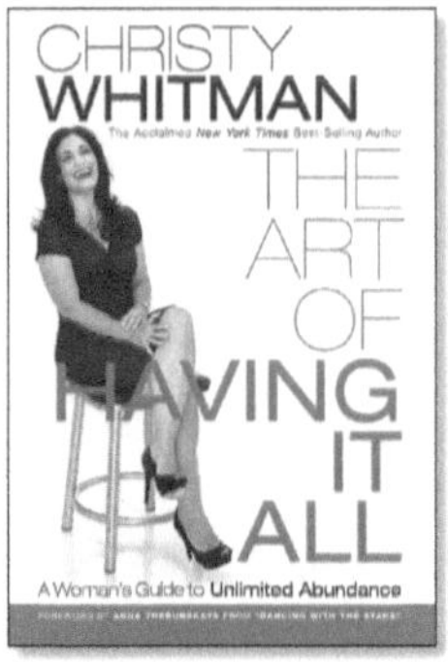

New York Times Best Seller
CHRISTY WHITMAN
The Art of Having It All: A Woman's Guide to Unlimited Abundance
Paperback: $16.95
Kindle/Nook: $9.99
Audible Book: $13.00

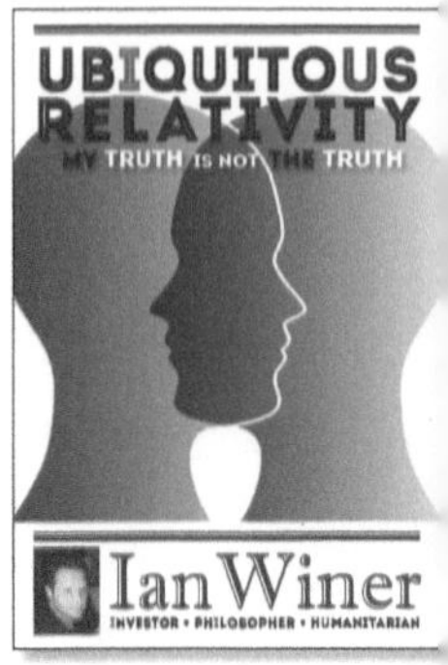

IAN WINER
Ubiquitous Relativity: My Truth is Not the Truth
Paperback: $16.95
Kindle: $9.99

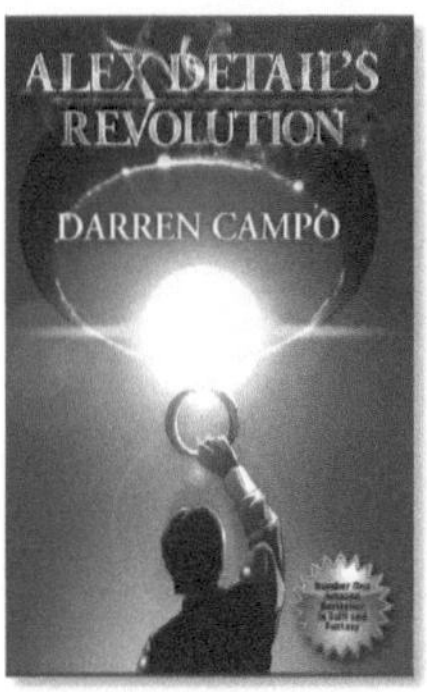

DARREN CAMPO
Alex Detail's Revolution
Paperback: $9.95
Hardcover: $22.95
Kindle: $9.15

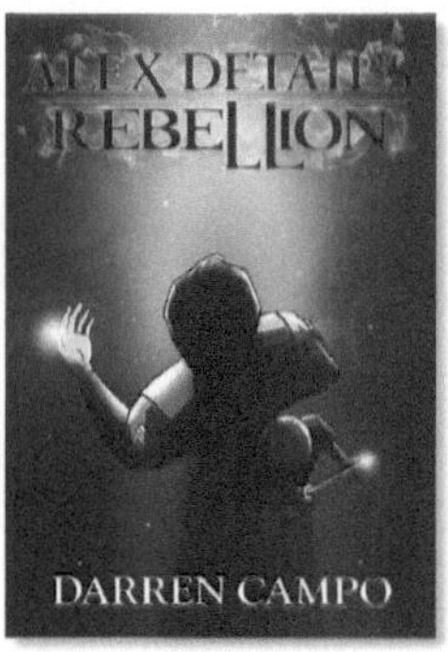

DARREN CAMPO
Alex Detail's Rebellion
Hardcover: $22.95
Kindle: $9.99

DARREN CAMPO
Disappearing Spell: Generationist Files: Book 1
Kindle: $2.99

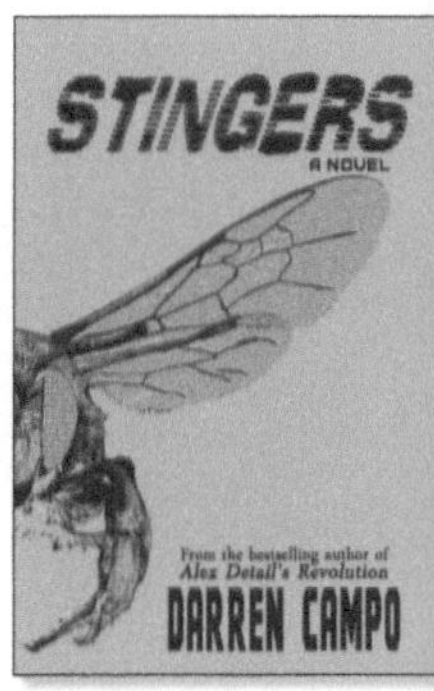

DARREN CAMPO
Stingers
Paperback: $9.99
Kindle: $9.99

TVGuestpert Publishing
11664 National Blvd, #345
Los Angeles, CA. 90064
310-584-1504
www.TVGPublishing.com

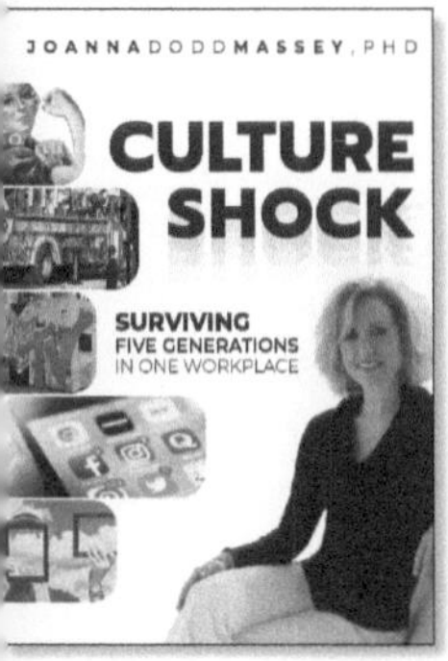

JOANNA DODD MASSEY
Culture Shock: Surviving Five Generations in One Workplace
Paperback: $16.95
Kindle/Nook: $9.99

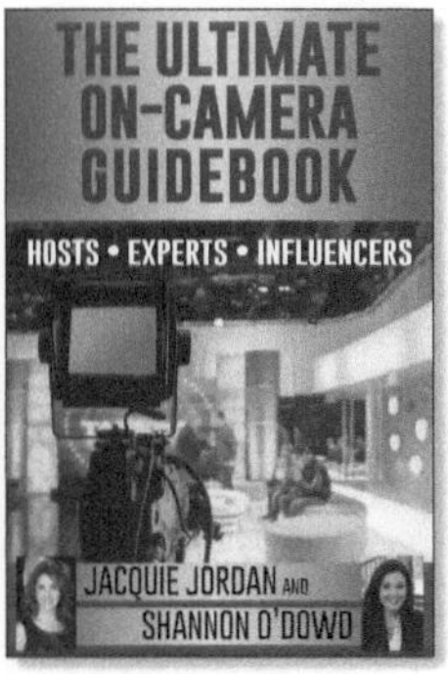

JACQUIE JORDAN AND SHANNON O'DOWD
*The Ultimate On-Camera Guidebook: Hosts*Experts*Influencers*
Paperback: $16.95
Kindle: $9.99

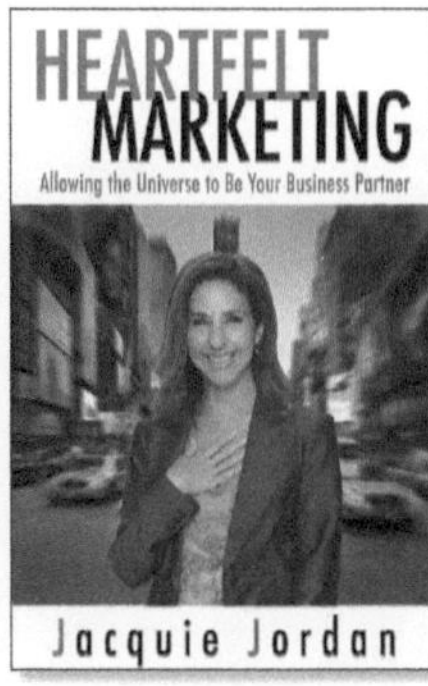

JACQUIE JORDAN
Heartfelt Marketing: Allowing the Universe to Be Your Business Partner
Paperback: $15.95
Kindle: $9.99
Audible: $9.95

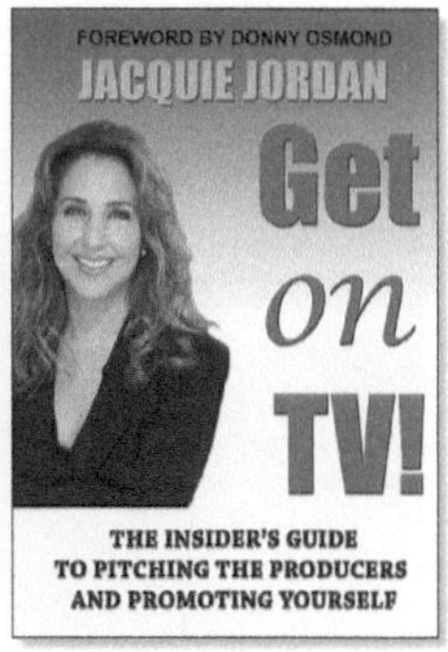

JACQUIE JORDAN
Get on TV! The Insider's Guide to Pitching the Producers and Promoting Yourself
Published by Sourcebooks
Paperback: $14.95
Kindle: $9.99
Nook: $14.95

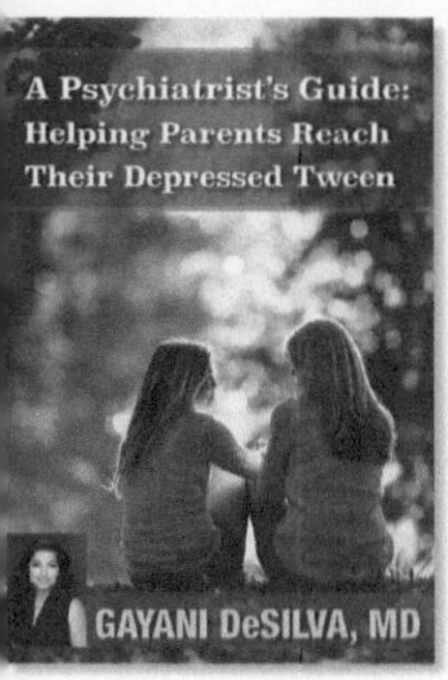

GAYANI DESILVA, MD
A Psychiatrist's Guide: Helping Parents Reach Their Depressed Tween
Paperback: $16.95
Kindle: $9.99

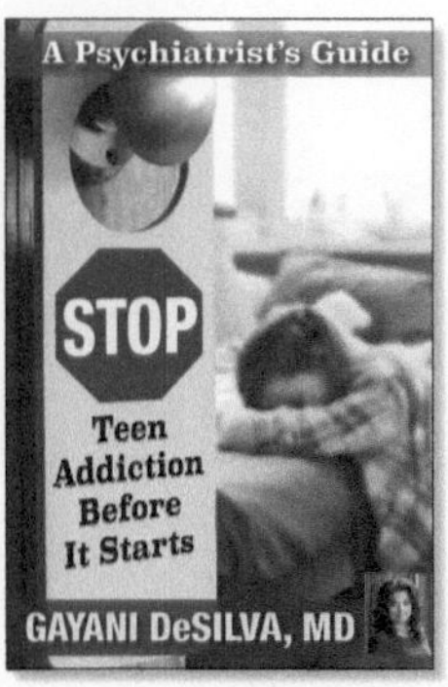

GAYANI DESILVA, MD
A Psychiatrist's Guide: Stop Teen Addiction Before It Starts
Paperback: $16.95
Kindle: $9.99
Audible: $14.95

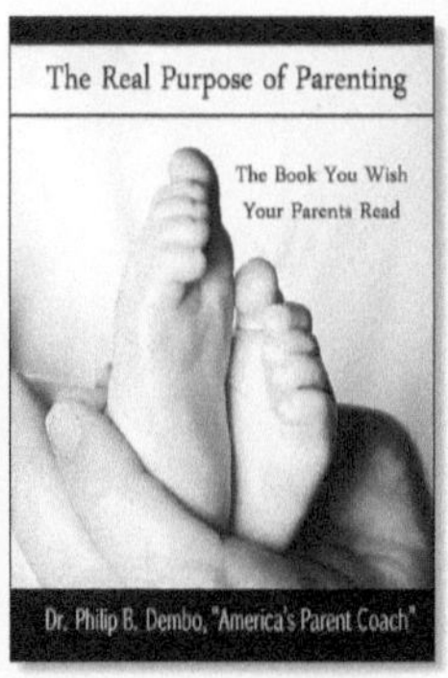

DR. PHILIP DEMBO
The Real Purpose of Parenting: The Book You Wish Your Parents Read
Paperback: $15.95
Kindle: $9.99
Audible: $23.95

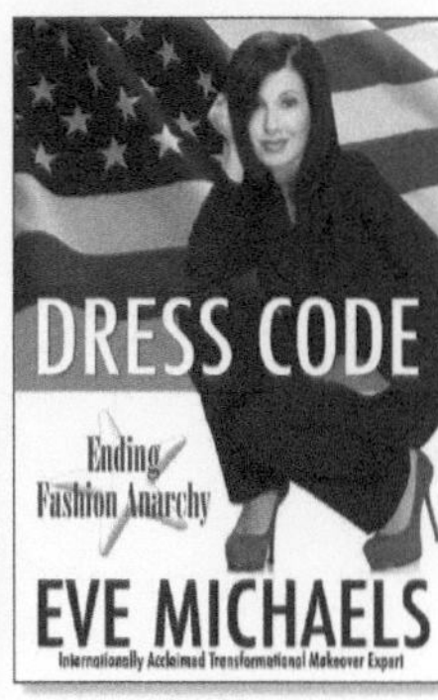

EVE MICHAELS
Dress Code: Ending Fashion Anarchy
Paperback: $15.95
Kindle/Nook: $9.99
Audible Book: $17.95

Published by

TVGUESTPERT PUBLISHING

TVGuestpert Publishing
11664 National Blvd, #34
Los Angeles, CA. 90064
310-584-1504
www.TVGPublishing.com

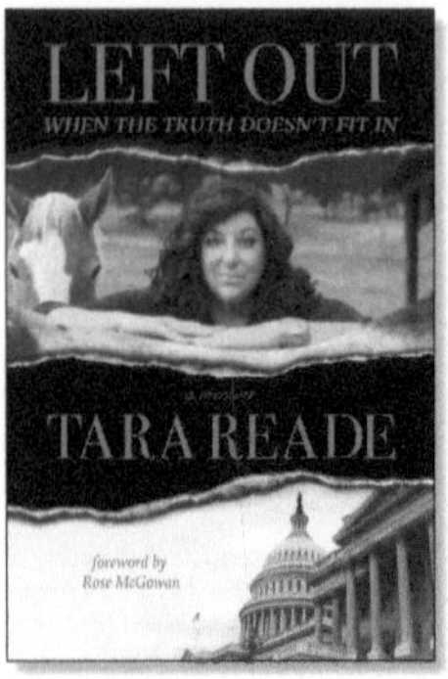

TARA READE
Left Out: When The Truth Doesn't Fit In
Hardcover: $22.95
Kindle: $9.99

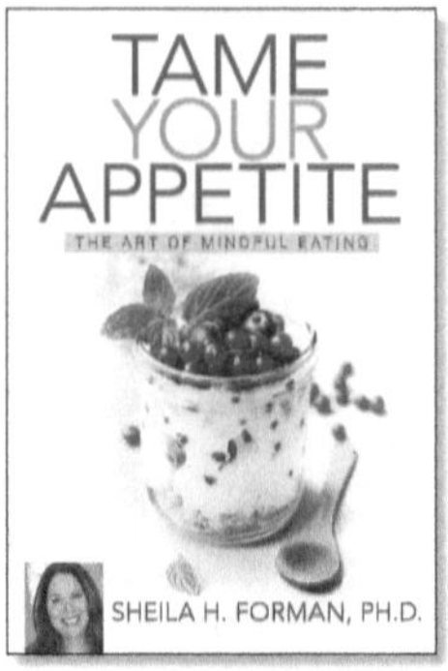

SHEILA H. FORMAN, Ph.D
Tame Your Appetite: The Art of Mindful Eating
Paperback: $16.95
Kindle: $9.99